RESPIRAT(

CASE STUDIES

THE THERAPIST-DRIVEN PROTOCOL APPROACH

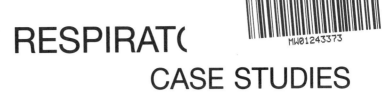

MW01243373

RESPIRATORY CARE
CASE STUDIES

THE THERAPIST-DRIVEN PROTOCOL APPROACH

TERRY DES JARDINS, M.Ed., R.R.T.

Director
Department of Respiratory Care
Parkland College
Champaign, Illinois

GEORGE G. BURTON, M.D., FACP, FCCP

Medical Director, Respiratory Services
Kettering Medical Center, Kettering, Ohio
Clinical Professor of Medicine and Anesthesiology
Wright State University School of Medicine
Dayton, Ohio

JUDITH TIETSORT, R.N., R.R.T.

Chairman
Respiratory Management Consultants
Arvada, Colorado

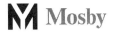 Mosby

St. Louis Baltimore Boston Carlsbad Chicago Naples New York Philadelphia Portland
London Madrid Mexico City Singapore Sydney Tokyo Toronto Wiesbaden

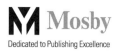

Mosby

Dedicated to Publishing Excellence

A Times Mirror Company

Vice President and Publisher: Don Ladig
Editor: Jennifer Roche
Developmental Editor: Anne Gleason
Project Manager: Patricia Tannian
Book Design Manager: Gail Morey Hudson
Manufacturing Supervisor: Karen Lewis
Cover Designer: Teresa Breckwoldt

Printed in the United States of America
Composition by Graphic World, Inc.
Printing/binding by Maple Vail Book Mfg. Group

Mosby–Year Book, Inc.
11830 Westline Industrial Drive
St. Louis, Missouri 63146

Photo credit: Figures 4-1, 8-1, 10-1, 11-1, 12-1, 17-1, 19-1, 23-1, 27-1, 28-1, and 29-1 are from Armstrong P, Wilson AG, Dee P. Hansel DM: *Imaging of Diseases of the Chest,* ed 2. St. Louis, 1995. Mosby–Year Book, Inc.

Library of Congress Cataloging in Publication Data

Des Jardins, Terry R.
    Respiratory care case studies: the therapist-driven protocol
approach / Terry Des Jardins, George Burton, Judy Tietsort.
       p.   cm.
    Includes bibliographical references and index.
    ISBN 0-8151-1366-8
    1. Respiratory therapy--Case studies. I. Burton, George G.,
1934–   . II. Tietsort, Judy. III. Title.
    [DNLM: 1. Respiratory Tract Diseases—therapy—case studies.
2. Respiratory Therapy—case studies.   WF 145 D441r 1996]
RC735.I5D4 1996
616.2′06—dc20
DNLM/DLC
for Library of Congress   96-23055
                                  CIP

96 97 98 99 00 / 9 8 7 6 5 4 3 2 1

To

JANE, JENNIFER, and MICHELLE

and to all the ***anonymous patients*** who provide

the foundation for the case study scenarios in this textbook.

TERRY

To

JEAN

who inspires, guides, and loves me,

and to my ***respiratory therapy students,*** who are

always one step ahead of me.

GEORGE

To my husband and daughters

ROD, BROOKE, and AMY

and to all the ***patients and respiratory therapy staff***

who over the years have made working in this field so rewarding.

JUDY

Preface

Delivering effective respiratory care requires critical thinking. Therefore, strong *assessment skills* are needed by any student coming up in the profession of respiratory care, as well as by the practitioner. *Respiratory Care Case Studies: The Therapist-Driven Protocol Approach* is designed to help respiratory care students learn when and how to assess patients, to challenge practitioners to build and perfect the assessment skills they use every day in clinical practice, and to guide managers through the successful implementation of a therapist-driven protocol (TDP) program.

Two pillars of the foundation of **strong assessment skills** include: (1) possession of a knowledge base of the major respiratory diseases and (2) competence in the performance of the assessment process. *Before the respiratory care practitioner is permitted to work unsupervised in a TDP program, training and competence in these two areas must be documented.*

Part I of this text provides an overview of the assessment process and knowledge base needed to perform successfully in a TDP environment. Parts II through XII present 29 case studies that ask the reader to gather important clinical data, write assessments, and select appropriate treatments. Following the case studies of six respiratory disorders that are most commonly encountered by respiratory care practitioners, key point questions are asked that challenge the reader to pinpoint fundamental concepts related to the specific respiratory disease.

Appendix I provides an answer key, including suggested responses for the case study assessment and treatment selections (SOAPs), thorough and thought-provoking discussion of each case, and answers to key point questions dealing with the six respiratory disorders most commonly treated by the respiratory therapist. Appendix II is an example of a respiratory assessment flow chart (SOAP) form.

ACKNOWLEDGMENTS

Shelly Mishoe, R.R.T., for allowing us to borrow and reformat her critical thinking format (for our Key Points sections) and for stimulating the respiratory care profession along the lines of problem-based learning.

Dee Johnson, M.S., R.R.T., for her help with the case of infant respiratory distress syndrome.

Deborah Beck, B.S., R.R.T., for her help in obtaining several chest radiographs for this book.

Terry Des Jardins
George G. Burton
Judith Tietsort

How to Use This Book

The purposes of this book are (1) to help students or practitioners expand their knowledge base and assessment skills independently and (2) to provide instructors or managers with a tool for teaching, evaluating, and documenting the competence of their students or staff in making assessments and treatment selections. These pages are perforated for the latter use.

Preceding the first assessment (SOAP)* completion form in each case are (1) the patient's admitting history, (2) clinical data related to the patient's initial physical examination, and (3) the specific respiratory therapy the patient is receiving. For example, the reader will be told "an arterial blood gas was obtained while the patient was receiving 2 L/min O_2 by nasal cannula." If the reader is not satisfied with the results of a selected therapy, he or she is expected to increase or decrease the therapy or to change it appropriately.

Readers are challenged to assess and treat the patients in this book by going through a thorough and systematic process of recording patient data. Several times within each case the reader is asked to create a problem-oriented medical record (POMR) for the patient, which includes the following information:

- The subjective and objective data collected from the patient
- An assessment based on the subjective and objective data
- The treatment plan (with measurable outcomes)

One of the most common POMR methods is the formulation of a SOAP progress note. SOAP is an acronym for 4 specific aspects of charting a patient's condition:

S: **Subjective** information refers to information provided by the patient about his or her feelings, concerns, or sensations. For example:

- "I coughed hard all night long."   • "My chest feels very tight."

Only the patient can provide subjective information. A comatose, intubated patient on a mechanical ventilator, therefore, would not be able to provide subjective data.

O: **Objective** information includes the data the respiratory care practitioner can measure, factually describe, or obtain from other clinical reports or test results. Objective data include the following:

- heart rate
- respiratory rate
- blood pressure
- temperature
- breath sounds
- cough effort
- sputum production (volume, consistency, color, and odor)
- arterial blood gas and pulse oximetry data
- pulmonary function study results
- x-rays
- hemodynamic data
- chemistry results

---

*Weed LL: *Medical record, medical education, and patient care: the problem-oriented record as a basic tool,* Cleveland, Ohio, 1971, Case Western Reserve University Press.

All the assessment answers in Appendix I are presented in the SOAP format: subjective, objective, assessment, and plan (see Fig. 1-2). For a more in-depth discussion of the SOAP format, see Des Jardins T, Burton GG: *Clinical manifestations and assessment of respiratory disease,* ed 3, St. Louis, 1995, Mosby.

A: **Assessment** refers to the practitioner's professional conclusion about what is the "cause" of the subjective and objective data presented by the patient. In a patient with a respiratory disorder the cause is most commonly due to a specific anatomic alteration of the lung. The assessment is the specific reason "why" the respiratory care practitioner is working with the patient. For example, the presence of wheezes would be objective data (the clinical indicator) to verify the assessment (the cause) of bronchial smooth muscle constriction; arterial blood gases—pH 7.18, $Paco_2$ 80 mm Hg, HCO_3^- 29 mmol/L, and Pao_2 54 mm Hg—would be the objective data to verify the assessment of acute ventilatory failure with moderate hypoxemia; or the presence of rhonchi would be a clinical indicator to verify the assessment of secretions in the large airways.

P: **Plan** is the therapeutic procedure(s) selected to remedy the cause identified in the assessment that is responsible for the subjective and objective data demonstrated by the patient. For example, an assessment of bronchial smooth muscle constriction would justify the administration of a bronchodilator; the assessment of acute ventilatory failure would justify mechanical ventilation.

   SOAP Example: A 26-year-old man presented in the emergency room with a severe asthmatic episode. On observation, his arms were fixed to the bed rails; he was using his accessory muscles of inspiration; and he was pursed-lip breathing. The patient stated that, "It feels like someone is standing on my chest. I just can't seem to take a deep breath." His heart rate was 111 bpm, and his blood pressure was 170/110. His respiratory rate was 28/min and shallow. Hyperresonant notes were produced upon percussion. Auscultation revealed expiratory wheezing and rhonchi bilaterally. His chest x-ray film revealed a severely depressed diaphragm and alveolar hyperinflation. His peak expiratory flow rate (PEFR) was 165 L/min. Even though his cough effort was weak, he produced a large amount of thick, white sputum. His arterial blood gases were pH 7.27, $Paco_2$ 62 mm Hg, HCO_3^-, 25 mmol/L, and Pao_2 49 mm Hg (on room air).

S "It feels like someone is standing on my chest. I can't take a deep breath."

O Uses accessory muscles of inspiration; pursed-lip breathing; hyperresonance; expiratory wheezing; depressed diaphragm and alveolor hyperinflation; PEFR 165; weak cough; large amount of thick, white sputum; pH 7.27; $Paco_2$ 62; HCO_3^- 25; Pao_2 49.

A Bronchospasm; hyperinflation; poor ability to mobilize thick secretions; acute ventilatory failure with severe hypoxemia.

P Bronchodilator treatment per protocol; CPT and PD per protocol; mucolytic per protocol; mechanical ventilation per protocol; ABGs q30min.

   After the treatment has been administered, another abbreviated SOAP note should be made to determine if the treatment plan needs to be "up-regulated" or "down-regulated." Because of the nature of this book, the patient will not always respond well to therapy—even when the reader has selected the appropriate therapy or follow-up therapy. For this reason, each case is discussed in detail (see discussion sections in Appendix I) and readers are further encouraged to discuss their treatment selections and possible patient outcomes with fellow students or therapists and with instructors or managers.

FOR USE IN AN ACADEMIC SETTING

Even with a strong knowledge base of the major respiratory disorders, the learner needs time and practice in carrying out the actual assessment process. Initially, this should be done in a controlled classroom environment. Ideally these sessions should be conducted after (or during) the presentation of each of the major respiratory disorders in the curriculum.

   During these practice sessions, students may work individually or in small groups on the cases presented in this book. It is recommended that each student or a representative from each group present the assessment(s) and treatment selection(s) to the rest of the class on a chalkboard or overhead projector. For example, the group representatives would go to the chalkboard (all at the same time) and write their assessment and treatment selection on the board.

The instructor should also have the students indicate (1) which specific treatment they have selected under a particular treatment protocol category (for example, incentive spirometry or continuous positive airway pressure under the hyperinflation therapy protocol) and (2) the intensity with which it is to be given (for example, treatment frequency b.i.d. or q.i.d.). This activity often serves as an excellent stimulus (for both the students and the instructor) to identify certain problems and to discuss acceptable assessments and treatment selections. Instructors who wish to present the cases in this book as testing exercises, rather than as review or homework, should remove the perforated pages in Appendix I on the first day of class.

FOR USE IN A CLINICAL SETTING

Ideally, two or more qualified assess-and-treat respiratory therapists should be involved in the evaluation and check-off process of respiratory clinical staff members (working to prove and document competency) or respiratory students (working on their clinical requirements). These qualified therapists could include the "Assessment" course instructor, key clinical instructors, respiratory care department heads, supervisors, or medical directors. All respiratory students and hospital staff members should at some time be required to put into writing (for documentation purposes) their success with several different patient assessment exercises, which could include the following:

1. Work through the cases in this book, disease by disease, without the benefit of the answers at the back (pages are perforated). Turn in "SOAPed" cases to clinical instructor or hospital supervisor.
2. Critically review and assess a past case. Did respiratory care do a good job? Did they do a bad job? Why or why not?
3. Write an assessment and treatment plan for several different patients throughout the hospital. A competent therapist will not need more than 10 or 15 minutes per case to complete this task.
4. Spend an entire day with the medical director. The student may be asked by the physician to provide a written assessment of and treatment plan for numerous patients around the hospital.

An assessment and treatment (SOAP) form (see Fig. 1-2 and Appendix II) is often helpful in both the classroom and clinical setting in the rapid collection and systematic organization of important clinical data, the formulation of an assessment, and the development of a treatment plan. The SOAP form provided may also be useful as a final testing tool and may be placed on file for documentation along with the SOAPed cases from this book. Such documentation should be updated periodically to validate the retention of assessment skills.

KEY POINTS FOR KEY DISEASES

A special feature—Key Points—has been added to enhance the reader's knowledge of those respiratory disorders that are most frequently encountered in the clinical setting: chronic bronchitis, asthma, pneumonia, pulmonary edema, adult respiratory distress syndrome, and postoperative atelectasis. The points that should be known and understood about these diseases are presented in the form of Key Point Questions. The question format, which is used to provoke the critical thinking ability that every respiratory care practitioner should use in assessment and treatment selection, follows this sequence:

1. **Basic Concept Formation** questions cover common knowledge and common sense information about the disorder. This section provides the

perception of the disorder that the lay person typically would have of the disease. Questions in this section may include the following in a patient with asthma: What are the general **anatomic alterations of the lungs** associated with the disorder (e.g., bronchospasm)? What are the common **causes** of the disorder (e.g., allergy to cat hair)? A person who has a brother or sister with asthma, for example, probably has more background knowledge about the disorder than the general public would have. The idea behind categorizing some concepts as basic is first to *recognize* the concepts and then to use them as a framework from which to build the data base in the next section.

2. **Advanced Data Base Formation** questions cover new and in-depth concepts the respiratory care practitioner should know and understand regarding the interrelationships of the **anatomic alterations of the lungs, pathophysiologic mechanisms, clinical manifestations,** and **treatment modalities.** Questions in this section might include the following: What is your image or vision of the anatomic alterations of the lungs associated with the respiratory disorder? (See Fig. 1-3 for an illustration of a three-component model of a prototype airway. Therapy may be directed to any or all components.) What pathophysiologic mechanisms are commonly activated as a result of the anatomic alterations of the lungs? What clinical manifestations are commonly activated as a result of the respiratory disorder?

3. **Assessment** questions cover information needed to assess and treat a patient with this disorder effectively. This section provides a more in-depth review of the clinical data presented in the case study, which in turn reflects the specific anatomic alterations of the lungs and the pathophysiologic mechanisms that are caused by the respiratory disorder. This section also looks at the issue of severity rating of the clinical manifestations presented by the patient. Questions in this section might include the following: In this case, which clinical manifestations support your assessment as to (1) your image of the anatomic alterations of the lungs and (2) the *pathophysiologic* mechanisms activated? Which specific clinical manifestations do you feel were the most important clinical indicators of the severity of the disorder?

4. **Application** questions cover what you can do to treat the patient's specific, identified problems. This section looks at the issue of selecting treatment protocols and modalities that will be the most effective in correcting or offsetting clinical manifestations caused by the anatomic alterations and pathophysiologic mechanisms associated with the disorder. Questions in this section could include the following: Based on the clinical data and your assessments, what treatment protocols are indicated in treating the problems identified? What are the advantages and disadvantages of the treatment modalities selected?

5. **Evaluation** questions cover the outcome analysis. This section includes the analysis of how the patient is responding to treatment. Questions in this section may include the following: What are the expected outcomes of each of the treatment protocols you selected? What should be monitored to determine how the patient is responding to the treatment modalities selected?

6. **Boundary Awareness** questions cover when and whom the practitioners should ask for help. Questions in this section might include the following: What signs indicate the patient's condition is approaching unsafe boundaries? At what point should a supervisor be asked for help? At what point should the patient's physician be called?

After studying the questions and answers in a Key Points section, the reader should be able to comfortably answer questions about the disorder (e.g., asthma or pneumonia) in general and the case in particular.

Contents

PART I
INTRODUCTION

1 **Assessments through Therapist-Driven Protocols,** 1

Introduction, 1
Knowledge base, 1
Assessment process, 3
Assessments commonly made by the respiratory care practitioner, 3
Treatment protocols commonly selected by the respiratory care practitioner, 4
Respiratory disorders commonly assessed in a TDP program, 7
Common anatomic alterations of the lungs, 8
Interrelationships between anatomic alterations of the lungs, pathophysiologic
   mechanisms, clinical manifestations, and treatment selections, 8

PART II
OBSTRUCTIVE AIRWAY DISEASES

2 **Chronic Bronchitis,** 17

Key point questions for chronic bronchitis, 22

3 **Emphysema,** 23

4 **Bronchiectasis,** 27

5 **Asthma,** 33

Key point questions for asthma, 38

6 **Cystic Fibrosis,** 39

7 **Croup Syndrome,** 45

PART III
INFECTIOUS PULMONARY DISEASES

8 **Pneumonia,** 51

Key point questions for pneumonia, 56

9 **Acquired Immunodeficiency Syndrome (AIDS),** 57

10 **Lung Abscess,** 61

11 **Tuberculosis,** 67

12 **Fungal Diseases of the Lungs,** 73

PART IV
PULMONARY VASCULAR DISEASES

13 **Pulmonary Edema,** 79

Key point questions for pulmonary edema, 84

14 **Pulmonary Embolism,** 85

PART V
CHEST AND PLEURAL TRAUMA

15 **Flail Chest,** 91

16 **Pneumothorax,** 97

PART VI
DISORDERS OF THE PLEURA AND CHEST WALL

17 **Pleural Disease,** 103

18 **Kyphoscoliosis,** 109

PART VII
ENVIRONMENTAL LUNG DISEASES

19 **Pneumoconiosis,** 115

PART VIII
NEOPLASTIC DISEASES

20 **Cancer of the Lungs,** 121

PART IX
DIFFUSE ALVEOLAR DISEASES

21 **Adult Respiratory Distress Syndrome,** 127

   Key point questions for adult respiratory distress syndrome, 132

22 **Idiopathic (infant) Respiratory Distress Syndrome,** 133

PART X
CHRONIC NONINFECTIOUS PARENCHYMAL DISEASES

23 **Chronic Interstitial Lung Disease,** 137

PART XI
NEUROLOGIC DISORDERS AND SLEEP APNEA

24 **Guillain-Barré Syndrome,** 143

25 **Myasthenia Gravis,** 147

26 **Sleep Apnea,** 151

PART XII
OTHER IMPORTANT TOPICS

27 **Near Drowning,** 155

28 **Smoke Inhalation and Thermal Injuries,** 161

29 **Postoperative Atelectasis,** 167

   Key point questions for postoperative atelectasis, 172

APPENDIX I
Suggested SOAP Responses, Case Discussions, and Key Point Answers, 173

2 Chronic Bronchitis, 173

   Key point answers for chronic bronchitis, 177

3 Emphysema, 179

4 Bronchiectasis, 181

5 Asthma, 183

Key point answers for asthma, 185

6 Cystic Fibrosis, 189

7 Croup Syndrome, 191

8 Pneumonia, 193

Key point answers for pneumonia, 195

9 Acquired Immunodeficiency Syndrome (AIDS), 197

10 Lung Abscess, 199

11 Tuberculosis, 201

12 Fungal Diseases of the Lungs, 203

13 Pulmonary Edema, 205

Key point answers for pulmonary edema, 207

14 Pulmonary Embolism, 209

15 Flail Chest, 211

16 Pneumothorax, 213

17 Pleural Disease, 215

18 Kyphoscoliosis, 217

19 Pneumoconiosis, 219

20 Cancer of the Lungs, 223

21 Adult Respiratory Distress Syndrome, 225

Key point answers for ARDS, 227

22 Idiopathic (infant) Respiratory Distress Syndrome, 229

23 Chronic Interstitial Lung Disease, 231

24 Guillain-Barré Syndrome, 233

25 Myasthenia Gravis, 235

26 Sleep Apnea, 237

27 Near Drowning, 239

28 Smoke Inhalation and Thermal Injuries, 241

29 Postoperative Atelectasis, 243

Key point answers for postoperative atelectasis, 245

APPENDIX II
SOAP Form, 249

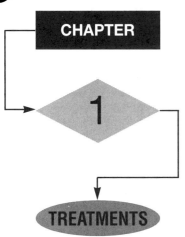

CHAPTER

1

TREATMENTS

Assessments Through Therapist-Driven Protocols

INTRODUCTION

Therapist-driven protocols (TDPs) have emerged as an integral part of respiratory care health services. TDPs provide much-needed flexibility to respiratory care practitioners and increase the quality of health care, as therapy can be more easily and efficiently modified according to the needs of the patient. TDPs are developed with input from physicians, and they are approved for use by the medical staff and the governing body of the hospitals in which they are used. Protocols give the respiratory care practitioner authority to evaluate the patient, initiate care, and to adjust, discontinue, or restart respiratory care procedures on a shift-by-shift, or hour-to-hour basis once the protocol is ordered by the physician.

In a good TDP program any one of the practitioners identified as TDP "safe and ready" can systematically gather the clinical data, formulate a correct assessment, and treat the patient appropriately and in essentially the same way any time of the day or year (Fig. 1-1, C). Clearly a strong TDP program promises a lot: that each therapist has a strong knowledge base of the respiratory disorders and competence in the actual assessment process. Fig. 1-1, B, illustrates how the strong knowledge base of the major respiratory disorders, the asessment process, and a good TDP program correlate with one another.

KNOWLEDGE BASE

The respiratory care practitioner with good assessment skills must first have a strong **knowledge base** of the major respiratory disorders. This knowledge base includes awareness of (1) the **anatomic alterations** of the lungs caused by common respiratory disorders, (2) the major **pathophysiologic mechanisms** activated throughout the respiratory system as a result of the anatomic alterations, (3) the common **clinical manifestations** that develop, and (4) the **treatment modalities** used to correct the anatomic alterations and pathophysiologic mechanisms caused by the disorder (Fig. 1-1, A).

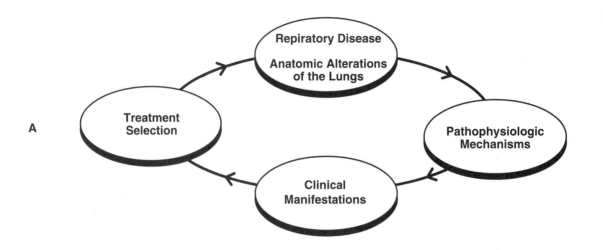

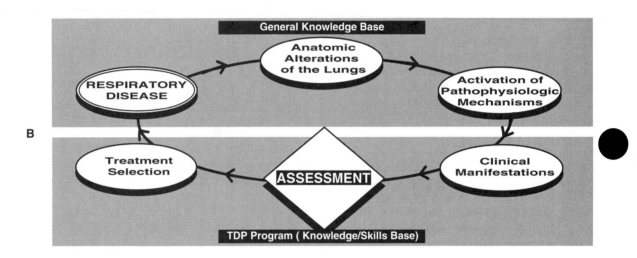

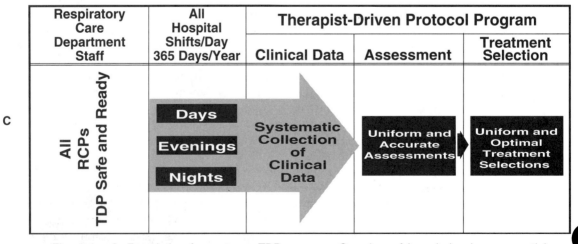

Fig. 1-1 **A,** Foundation for a strong TDP program. Overview of knowledge base essential for assessment of respiratory diseases. **B,** How knowledge, assessment, and TDP program interface. **C,** The promise of a good TDP program.

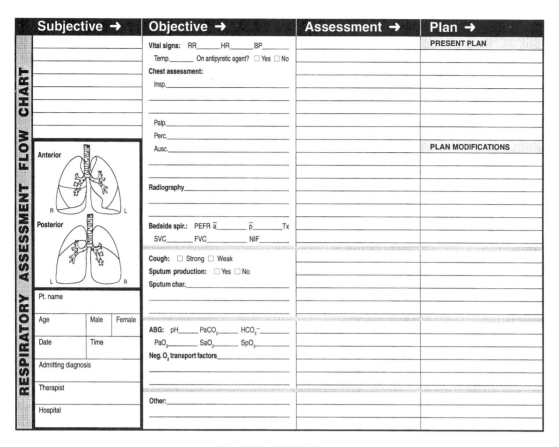

Fig. 1-2   SOAP form.

ASSESSMENT PROCESS

The respiratory care practitioner with good assessment skills must also be competent in performing the actual **assessment process.** This means the practitioner can (1) quickly and systematically collect the important clinical manifestations demonstrated by the patient, (2) formulate an accurate assessment of the clinical data, that is, identify the causes and severity of the data abnormalities, (3) select an optimal treatment modality, and (4) **document** this process quickly and in a clear and precise manner. For the new practitioner a predesigned SOAP form (Fig. 1-2 and Appendix II) is often used to facilitate the (1) rapid collection and systematic organization of important clinical data, (2) formulation of an assessment, and (3) selection of a treatment plan.

ASSESSMENTS COMMONLY MADE BY THE RESPIRATORY CARE PRACTITIONER

Immediately after the respiratory care practitioner systematically collects and documents the appropriate clinical data, an *assessment* must be formulated. For the most part the assessments formulated by the respiratory care practitioner are directed at the following objectives.

1. Identification of the specific **anatomic alterations of the lungs,** which activate specific *pathophysiologic mechanisms,* which in turn lead to specific *clinical manifestations*
2. Developing a **severity index** of the clinical manifestation(s) demonstrated by the patient, for example, a disabling cough effort or impending ventilatory failure

The table on p. 5 provides assessments commonly made by the respiratory care practitioner. For example, according to the assessments presented in the table an appropriate assessment for the clinical manifestation of wheezing might be bronchospasm. If the practitioner assesses the cause of the wheezing correctly, the appropriate treatment plan can be selected easily, in this case, *Bronchodilator Therapy Protocol,* to offset the anatomic alteration of bronchospasm. However, if the cause of the wheezing was correctly assessed to be excessive airway secretions, the appropriate treatment plan would entail a specific treatment modality under the *Bronchial Hygiene Therapy Protocol.*

TREATMENT PROTOCOLS COMMONLY SELECTED BY THE RESPIRATORY CARE PRACTITIONER

The treatment portion of a TDP, or respiratory care protocol, is based on selection of treatment procedures that will work best to correct or offset the anatomic alterations and pathophysiologic mechanisms caused by the respiratory disorder.

It should be emphasized that the treatment portion of a protocol, commonly referred to as a specific *treatment protocol* (for example, Oxygen Therapy Protocol or Hyperinflation Therapy Protocol), is only a part of a TDP. Before a specific treatment protocol can be administered, objective data and a correct assessment justifying the therapy *must* first be secured and documented (see Fig. 1-1, *C*).

In addition, it should be understood that the *precise treatment selected* (under a general treatment protocol category) and the *frequency* or *intensity* with which the treatment selection is administered are based primarily on the following:

1. Severity of the clinical manifestations demonstrated by the patient
2. Patient's ability to perform or tolerate the therapy

For example, a general treatment protocol category to prevent or correct atelectasis after thoracic surgery is the Hyperinflation Therapy Protocol. More precisely, however, if the patient is unconscious or unable to follow directions, a continuous positive airway pressure (CPAP) mask might be a more appropriate treatment selection (under the Hyperinflation Therapy Protocol) than, say, incentive spirometry, even though both are designed to treat or prevent atelectasis.

Treatment Protocol Categories: The Top Four

The foundation of a successful TDP program is composed of four treatment protocols: Oxygen Therapy Protocol, Hyperinflation Therapy Protocol, Bronchial Hygiene Therapy Protocol, and Bronchodilator Therapy Protocol. Common treatment selections from these protocols are listed in the boxes on pp. 6 and 7.

It should be understood that under each treatment protocol there are usually several different treatment modalities (officially approved by the medical staff and administration) that the respiratory care practitioner may select and administer to the patient to achieve the same therapeutic goal, for example, to increase the patient's oxygenation status to within a predetermined range (see boxes on pp. 6 and 7).

Finally, it should be noted that even when the patient is transferred to the intensive care unit and placed on a mechanical ventilator it is usually still necessary to administer one or more of the top four respiratory care treatment protocols. For example, the Hyperinflation Therapy Protocol via CPAP.

ASSESSMENTS
and Treatment Selections Commonly Made by the Respiratory Care Practitioner

OBJECTIVE CLINICAL DATA (examples)	ASSESSMENTS (cause of objective clinical data)	PLAN (physician ordered[†]) (common treatment selections)
Vital signs		
↑breathing rate, ↑blood pressure, ↑pulse	Respiratory distress	Treat underlying cause
Airways		
Wheezing	Bronchospasm	Bronchodilator Tx
Inspiratory stridor	Laryngeal edema	Cool mist
Rhonchi	Secretions in large airways	Bronchial hygiene Tx
Crackles	Secretions in distal airways	Treat underlying cause — e.g., CHF Hyperinflation Tx
Cough		
Strong cough	Good ability to mobilize secretions	None
Weak cough	Poor ability to mobilize secretions	Bronchial hygiene Tx
Secretions		
Amount: > 30 ml/24 hrs.	Excessive bronchial secretions	Bronchial hygiene Tx
White and translucent sputum	Normal sputum	None
Yellow/opaque sputum	Acute airway infection	Treat underlying cause
Green sputum	Old, retained secretions and infections	Bronchial hygiene Tx
Brown sputum	Old blood	Bronchial hygiene Tx
Red sputum	Fresh blood	Notify physician
Frothy secretions	Pulmonary edema	Treat underlying cause — e.g., CHF Hyperinflation Tx
Alveoli		
Bronchial breath sounds	Atelectasis	
Dull percussion note	Infiltrates	Hyperinflation Tx, oxygen Tx
Opacity on chest x-ray	Fibrosis	
Restrictive PFT values	Consolidation	No specific, effective respiratory care Tx
Depressed diaphragm on x-ray	Airtrapping and hyperinflation	Treat underlying cause
Pleural space		
Hyperresonant percussion note	Pneumothorax	Evacuate air[†] and hyperinflation Tx
Dull percussion note	Pleural effusion	Evacuate fluid[†] and hyperinflation Tx
Thorax		
Paradoxical movement of the chest wall	Flail chest	Mechanical ventilation[†]
Barrel chest	Airtrapping (hyperinflation)	Treat underlying cause — e.g., asthma
Posterior and lateral curvature of spine	Kyphoscoliosis	Bronchial hygiene Tx
Arterial Blood Gases — Ventilatory		
pH ↑, $PaCO_2$ ↓, HCO_3 ↓	Acute alveolar hyperventilation	Treat underlying cause
pH N, $PaCO_2$ ↓, HCO_3 ↓↓	Chronic alveolar hyperventilation	Generally none
pH ↓, $PaCO_2$ ↑, HCO_3 ↑	Acute ventilatory failure	Mechanical ventilation[†]
pH N, $PaCO_2$ ↑, HCO_3 ↑↑	Chronic ventilatory failure	Low flow oxygen, bronchial hygiene
Sudden Ventilatory Changes on Chronic Ventilatory Failure (CVF)		
pH ↑, $PaCO_2$ ↑, HCO_3 ↑↑, PaO_2 ↓	Acute alveolar hyperventilation on CVF	Treat underlying cause
pH ↓, $PaCO_2$ ↑↑, HCO_3 ↑, PaO_2 ↓	Acute ventilatory failure on CVF	Mechanical ventilation[†]
Metabolic		
pH ↑, $PaCO_2$ N or ↑, HCO_3 ↑, PaO_2 N	Metabolic alkalosis	Give potassium[†] — Hypokalemia Give chloride[†] — Hypochloremia
pH ↓, $PaCO_2$ N or ↓, HCO_3 ↓, PaO_2 ↓	Metabolic acidosis	Give oxygen — Lactic acidosis
pH ↓, $PaCO_2$ N or ↓, HCO_3 ↓, PaO_2 N	Metabolic acidosis	Give insulin[†] — Ketoacidosis
pH ↓, $PaCO_2$ N or ↓, HCO_3 ↓, PaO_2 N	Metabolic acidosis	Renal therapy[†]
Indication For Mechanical Ventilation		
pH ↑, $PaCO_2$ ↓, HCO_3 ↓, PaO_2 ↓	Impending ventilatory failure	
pH ↓, $PaCO_2$ ↑, HCO_3 ↑, PaO_2 ↓	Ventilatory failure	Mechanical ventilation[†]
pH ↓, $PaCO_2$ ↑, HCO_3 ↑, PaO_2 ↓	Apnea	
Oxygenation Status		
PaO_2 < 80 mm Hg	Mild hypoxemia	
PaO_2 < 60 mm Hg	Moderate hypoxemia	Oxygen Tx and treat underlying cause
PaO_2 < 40 mm Hg	Severe hypoxemia	
Oxygen Transport Status		
↓ PaO_2, anemia, ↓ cardiac output	Inadequate oxygen transport	Oxygen Tx and treat underlying cause

OXYGEN THERAPY PROTOCOL

OBJECTIVE

To Treat Hypoxemia, Decrease the Work of Breathing, or Decrease Myocardial Work

Common treatment modalities

- Nasal cannula
- Oxygen mask
- Venturi mask
- Partial rebreathing mask
- Nonrebreathing mask

HYPERINFLATION THERAPY PROTOCOL

OBJECTIVE

To Prevent or Treat Alveolar Consolidation and Atelectasis

Common treatment modalities

- Cough and deep breathing (C & DB)
- Incentive spirometry (IS)
- Intermittent positive-pressure breathing (IPPB)
- Continuous positive airway pressure (CPAP)
- Positive end-expiratory pressure (PEEP)

BRONCHIAL HYGIENE THERAPY PROTOCOL

OBJECTIVE

To Enhance Mobilization of Bronchial Secretions

Common treatment modalities

- Increased bronchial hydration
  - Increased fluid intake (6-10 glasses of water a day)
  - Bland aerosol therapy
  - Ultrasonic nebulization (USN)
- Cough and deep breathing (C & DB)
  - Techniques used to enhance cough and deep breathing
    - Incentive spirometry (IS)
    - Intermittent positive-pressure breathing (IPPB)
    - Positive expiratory pressure (PEP) therapy
- Chest physical therapy (CPT)
- Postural drainage (PD)
- Percussion and vibration with postural drainage
- Suctioning
- Mucolytic therapy
  - Acetylcysteine (Mucomyst)
  - Recombinant human DNase (rhDNase) (Pulmozyme)
  - Sodium bicarbonate (2% solution)
- Assist physician in bronchoscopy

BRONCHODILATOR THERAPY PROTOCOL

OBJECTIVE
To Induce Bronchial Smooth Muscle Relaxation

Common treatment modalities
e.g., via metered dose inhaler (MDI), hand-held nebulizer, or intermittent positive-pressure breathing (IPPB)

- Sympathomimetic bronchodilator therapy
  - Metaproterenol (Alupent or Metaprel)
  - Albuterol (Proventil or Ventolin)
  - Terbutaline (Brethine or Brethaire)
- Parasympatholytic bronchodilator therapy
  - Atropine sulfate
  - Ipratropium bromide (Atrovent)

RESPIRATORY DISORDERS COMMONLY ASSESSED IN A TDP PROGRAM

Although the respiratory care practitioner may treat at least one or two cases of every disorder presented in this text, most of the respiratory care practitioner's professional career will be spent caring for only a few of them. It is estimated that as much as 80% of the respiratory care practitioner's work is concerned with the intelligent assessment and treatment selection of a short list of respiratory illnesses (see table below).

Common Respiratory Disorders

Respiratory Disorder	DRG Number*
OBSTRUCTIVE	
Chronic bronchitis	88
Emphysema	88
Asthma	98
Combination of all three	—
RESTRICTIVE	
Pneumonia	89
Atelectasis	101/102
Adult respiratory distress syndrome	99/100
Pulmonary edema	87

Respiratory disorders can be identified by their respective diagnosis-related group or DRG. DRG is an identificaton system used to categorize and document diseases, primarily for use in health care reimbursement (such as Medicaid and Medicare). Patients are routinely assigned to a DRG based on their admitting diagnosis, and each DRG has its own identifying number. DRGs are also commonly used to document and communicate information about patients. Because the use of DRGs is prevalent, it is important for respiratory care practitioners to recognize and understand the DRGs they will commonly encounter.

COMMON ANATOMIC ALTERATIONS OF THE LUNG

The respiratory disorders listed in the preceding table represent the common anatomic alterations of the lungs treated by the respiratory care practitioner. The major anatomic alterations include (1) **atelectasis** (e.g., following upper thoracic surgery), (2) **consolidation** (e.g., pneumonia), (3) **increased alveolar-capillary membrane thickness** (e.g., adult respiratory distress syndrome [ARDS], pulmonary edema), (4) **bronchospasm** (e.g., asthma), (5) **excessive bronchial secretions** (e.g., bronchitis, asthma, or pulmonary edema), and (6) **distal airway and alveolar weakening** (e.g., emphysema).

INTERRELATIONSHIPS BETWEEN ANATOMIC ALTERATIONS OF THE LUNGS, PATHOPHYSIOLOGIC MECHANISMS, CLINICAL MANIFESTATIONS, AND TREATMENT SELECTIONS

Specific *anatomic alterations* of the lung (such as those just listed) activate specific, predictable *pathophysiologic mechanisms.* Common pathophysiologic mechanisms activated in respiratory diseases are listed in the box below. The pathophysiologic mechanisms, in turn, activate specific, predictable *clinical manifestations* (see Fig. 1-1, *C*).

Thus when the common interrelationships between the major anatomic alterations of the lungs, the pathophysiologic mechanisms, and the clinical manifestations are known and understood by the respiratory care practitioner, the appropriate treatment protocol can easily be selected. Fig. 1-3, a three-component model of a prototype airway, is helpful in visualizing the anatomic alterations of the lungs commonly associated with respiratory disorders. To further enhance the student's understanding of these important interrelationships, review Figs. 1-4 to 1-9.

PATHOPHYSIOLOGIC MECHANISMS COMMONLY ACTIVATED IN RESPIRATORY DISORDERS

- Decreased ventilation/perfusion ($\dot{V}/\dot{Q}$) ratio
- Alveolar diffusion block
- Decreased lung compliance
- Stimulation of oxygen receptors
- Deflation reflex
- Irritant reflex
- Pulmonary reflex
- Increased airway resistance
- Air trapping and alveolar hyperinflation

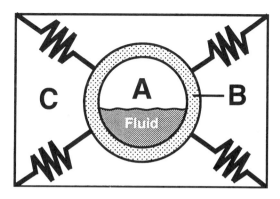

Fig. 1-3   A three-component model of a prototype airway. Therapy may be directed to any or all components. *A* = airway lumen, *B* = airway wall, *C* = supporting structures. Therapy for *A:* Deep breathing and coughing, smoking cessation, suctioning, mucolytics, bland aerosols, systemic and parenteral hydration, therapeutic bronchoscopy. Therapy for *B:* Bronchodilators, aerosolized anti-inflammatory agents, aerosolized antibiotics, aerosolized decongestants. Therapy for *C:* Pursed-lip breathing exercises and removal of external factors compressing the airway (bullae, pleural effusion, pneumothorax, tumor masses).

Key to abbreviations in Figs. 1-4 to 1-9, pp. 10 to 15:

ABG   = arterial blood gases
ARDS = adult respiratory distress syndrome
CPAP = continuous positive airway pressure
CPT   = chest physical therapy
Do_2 = total oxygen delivery
ERV   = expiratory reserve volume
FEF   = forced expiratory flow, midexpiratory phase
FEV_1 = forced expiratory volume in 1 second
FEVT = forced expiratory volume (timed)
FRC   = functional residual capacity
FVC   = forced vital capacity
IC   = inspiratory capacity
MVV   = maximum voluntary ventilation
O_2ER = oxygen extraction ratio
PD   = postural drainage
PEEP = positive end-expiratory pressure
PEFR = peak expiratory flow rate
PFT   = pulmonary function test
$\dot{Q}s/\dot{Q}_T$ = cardiac output shunted/total cardiac output
RV   = residual volume
$S\bar{v}o_2$ = mixed venous oxygen saturation
TLC   = total lung capacity
VC   = vital capacity
$\dot{V}/\dot{Q}$ = ventilation/perfusion

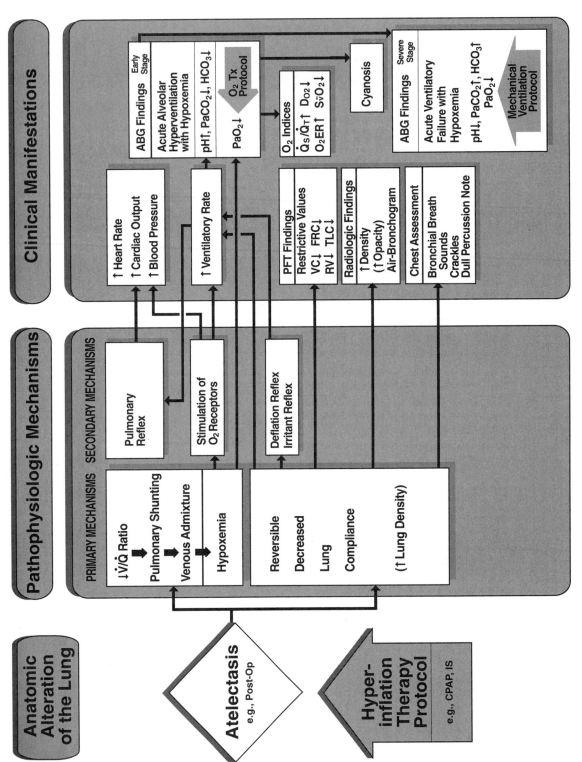

Fig. 1-4   The hypoxemia that develops as a result of atelectasis is caused by capillary shunting. Hypoxemia caused by capillary shunting is refractory to oxygen therapy. Thus implementation of the Hyperinflation Therapy Protocol may be more beneficial in the treatment of this hypoxemia than the Oxygen Therapy Protocol would be.

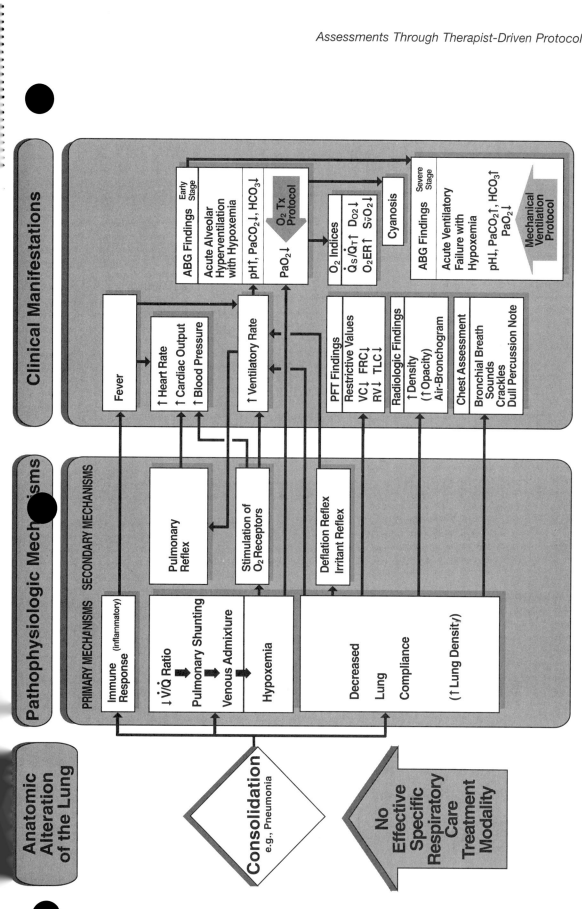

Fig. 1-5   The hypoxemia due to alveolar consolidation is caused by capillary shunting. Hypoxemia due to capillary shunting is refractory to oxygen therapy. There is no effective, specific respiratory care treatment modality for alveolar consolidation. With pneumonia the great temptation for the respiratory care practitioner is to do too much, such as hyperinflation therapy, bronchodilator therapy, and bronchial hygiene therapy. Such treatment protocols generally are not indicated, especially during the early stages. With pneumonia, appropriate antibiotics (prescribed by the physician), bedrest, fluids, and supplementary oxygen are all that is needed. When pneumonia is in its resolution stage, however, there may be excessive secretions and atelectasis, accompanied by bronchoconstriction. At this time, other treatment modalities may be indicated.

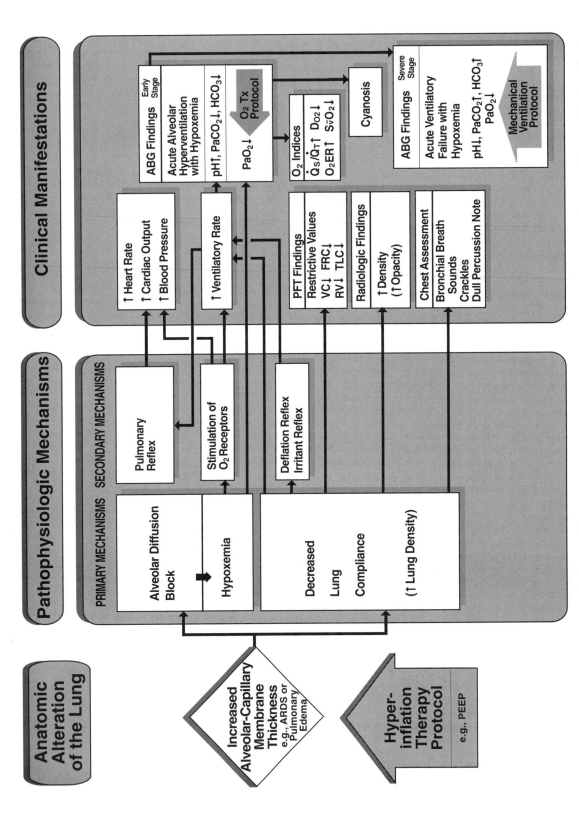

Fig. 1-6 The hypoxemia that develops as a result of an increased alveolar-capillary membrane thickness is caused by an alveolar diffusion block. Hypoxemia caused by a diffusion block often responds favorably to oxygen therapy.

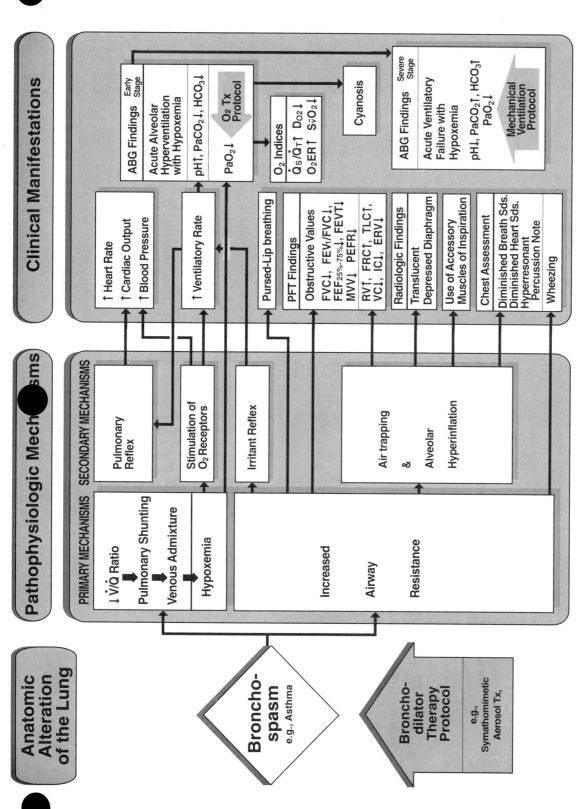

Fig. 1-7   The *Bronchodilator Therapy Protocol* is the primary treatment modality used to offset the anatomic alteration of bronchospasm (the original cause of the pathophysiologic chain of events); the *Oxygen Therapy Protocol* and the *Mechanical Ventilation Protocol* are secondary treatment modalities used to offset the mild, moderate, or severe clinical manifestations associated with bronchospasm. When the patient responds favorably to the Bronchodilator Therapy Protocol, the need for the Oxygen Therapy Protocol may be minimal and for the Mechanical Ventilation Protocol not at all.

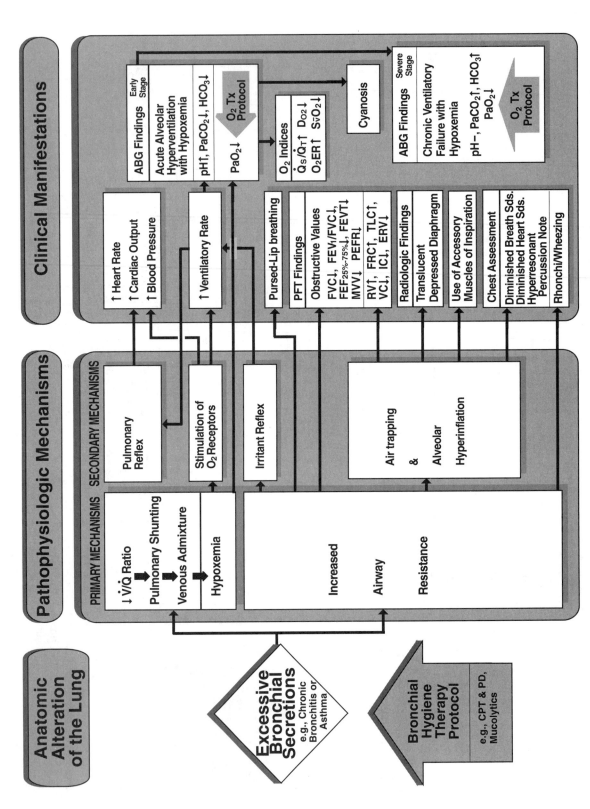

Fig. 1-8 The Bronchial Hygiene Therapy Protocol is the primary treatment modality used to offset excessive bronchial secretions. Note that when the patient demonstrates chronic ventilatory failure during the advanced stages of chronic bronchitis, caution must be taken with the Oxygen Therapy Protocol not to eliminate the patient's hypoxic ventilatory drive.

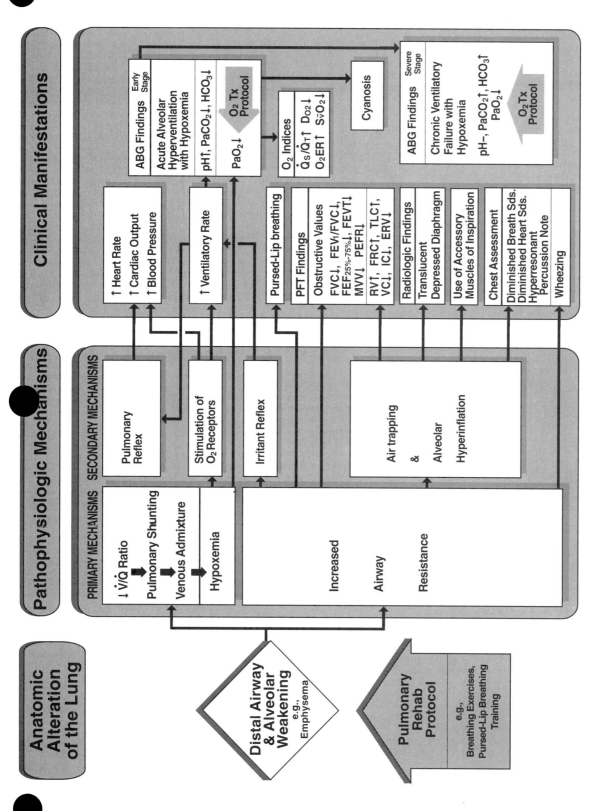

Fig. 1-9   Pulmonary rehabilitation and oxygen therapy may be all that can be done to treat distal airway and alveolar weakening. Note that when the patient demonstrates chronic ventilatory failure during the advanced stage of emphysema, caution must be taken with the Oxygen Therapy Protocol not to eliminate the patient's hypoxic ventilatory drive.

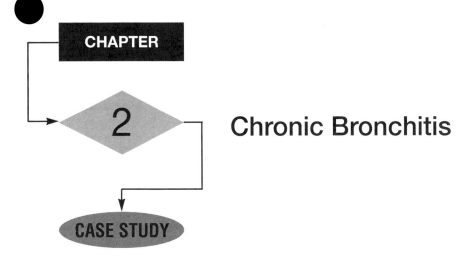

CHAPTER

2

CASE STUDY

Chronic Bronchitis

ADMITTING HISTORY

This 68-year-old retired geologist arrived in the emergency room with his daughter. He was well known to the respiratory care consult team. He had a 40-year history of smoking a pack of cigarettes a day, was widowed, lived alone, and had difficulty managing his daily activities. For the past week the patient had experienced increased dyspnea and cough and had been unable to care for himself. On observation it was obvious his personal hygiene had deteriorated. The patient stated that he was unable to get his breath or to inhale deep enough to cough up secretions. He complained of mild nausea without abdominal pain or vomiting.

The patient had been diagnosed with severe chronic bronchitis approximately 6 years ago and had had an acute myocardial infarction 2 years ago. His pulmonary function studies 1 year before this admission showed severe airway obstruction and air trapping. He had a history of high blood pressure, congestive heart failure, chronic dyspnea on exertion, chronic cough, and two episodes of pneumonia within the last year. In recent months, according to a neighbor, he had become increasingly depressed.

According to his daughter his physical activity was minimal. He generally spent most of his days watching television, smoking, and napping. All his children, none of whom lived in the immediate area, had been trying to coax him to move to a boarding house environment, but he adamantly refused. During his last admission the advantages of pulmonary rehabilitation were discussed with him. The patient felt he had no need for pulmonary education as well as no need for other agencies or organizations to check up on him in his home.

PHYSICAL EXAMINATION (Time: 1730)

Inspection revealed a barrel chest, clubbing of his fingers and toes, cyanotic skin, and 1+ pitting edema around his ankles. His breathing was labored; he was pursed-lip breathing, using his accessory muscles of respiration, and he appeared weak. He had a frequent, weak cough productive of large amounts of thick, yellow sputum.

Vital signs were blood pressure 190/115, heart rate 125 bpm, respiratory rate 30/min, and temperature 37° C (98.6° F). Tactile fremitus was present over both lung fields, and hyperresonant percussion notes were produced both anteriorly and posteriorly. Bilateral rhonchi were auscultated. His abdomen was soft and was not tender. Bowel sounds were active.

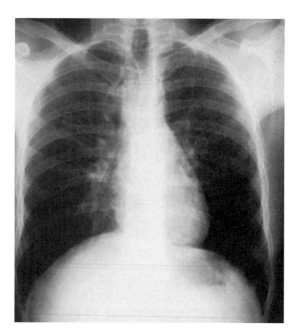

Fig. 2-1

On room air his arterial blood gas values were pH 7.53, Pa_{CO_2} 56 mm Hg, HCO_3^- 33 mmol/L, and Pa_{O_2} 43 mm Hg. Review of his chart showed that on his last hospital discharge his baseline arterial blood gas values on 2 L/min O_2 were pH 7.39, Pa_{CO_2} 85 mm Hg, HCO_3^- 38 mmol/L, and Pa_{O_2} 64 mm Hg. His carboxyhemoglobin level was 6%. His chest x-ray film on this admission showed severe air trapping and depressed hemidiaphragms. No acute infiltrates were seen. His heart size was normal (Fig. 2-1). His complete blood count values were all normal except for a hematocrit of 58%. The attending physician ordered a respiratory care consult. This was written in the patient's chart: "All efforts should be made to keep the patient off the ventilator."

RESPONSE 1

On the basis of the above information, write your SOAP in the following space.

S _____

_____

O _____

_____

_____

_____

_____

_____

_____

_____

A _____
_____
_____
_____
_____
_____
_____
_____
_____

P _____
_____
_____
_____
_____
_____

EARLY MORNING, NEXT DAY (Time: 0230)

The respiratory care practitioner on duty was called by the floor nurse to evaluate the patient. The nurse reported that the patient said that he was having a bad period. The nurse further felt that the patient appeared restless and short of breath and was coughing excessively.

On inspection the patient could be seen using his accessory muscles of respiration; he demonstrated pursed-lip breathing. He demonstrated a weak, productive cough. He expectorated large amounts of thick, yellow secretions. The patient's vital signs were blood pressure 185/135, heart rate 130 bpm, respiratory rate 28/min, and temperature 37° C (98.6° F). Bilateral rhonchi were auscultated over the lung bases. His arterial blood gas values were pH 7.55, $Paco_2$ 53 mm Hg, HCO_3^- 32 mmol/L, Pao_2 41 mm Hg. His hemoglobin oxygen saturation measured by pulse oximetry (SpO_2) was 83%.

RESPONSE 2

On the basis of the above information, write your SOAP in the following space.

S _____

O _____
_____
_____
_____
_____

A _____

_____

_____

_____

_____

_____

_____

P _____

_____

_____

_____

_____

LATE AFTERNOON, SAME DAY (Time: 1415)

Although the patient had been resting comfortably for several hours, he suddenly became short of breath and difficult to arouse just before a scheduled bronchial hygiene treatment. The respiratory therapist on duty noted that the patient said that he was "doing worse again." He was sitting up in bed and using his accessory muscles of respiration and pursed-lip breathing. His breathing was rapid and shallow. His cough continued to be weak. No sputum production was noted at this time. Expiration was prolonged.

The patient's vital signs were blood pressure 150/95, heart rate 140 bpm, respiratory rate 25/min, and temperature normal. He had bilateral rhonchi. A recent chest x-ray film was not available. His arterial blood gas values were pH 7.28, Pa_{CO_2} 105 mm Hg, HCO_3^- 41 mmol/L, and Pa_{O_2} 44 mm Hg. His carboxyhemoglobin level was 2.5%. A toxic drug blood screen was negative.

RESPONSE 3

On the basis of the above information, write your SOAP in the following space.

S _____

_____

O _____

_____

_____

_____

A

P

➥ KEY POINT QUESTIONS | *For Chronic Bronchitis (DRG 88)*

1. **Basic Concept Formation**
   a. What is the most common *cause* of chronic bronchitis?
   b. Are the *clinical manifestations* of cough and sputum production characteristic of this disorder? If so, why?
   c. How are secretions normally *cleared* from the airway?
   d. Are these mechanisms impaired in patients with chronic bronchitis?
   e. Does *smoking cessation* improve the symptoms of chronic bronchitis?
2. **Data Base Formation**
   a. What is your *vision* of the pathology of chronic bronchitis?
   b. What *pathophysiologic mechanisms* are activated as a result of the typical anatomic alterations?
   c. What portion(s) of the *airway model* (see Fig. 1-3) is/are abnormal in chronic bronchitis?
   d. What are the *extrapulmonary signs and symptoms* of severe cases of chronic bronchitis?
   e. What should be the *goals of therapy* for such patients?
   f. Which *standard TDPs* would achieve these goals?
   g. What are the expected *outcomes,* possible *adverse effects,* and *monitors* of the beneficial and adverse effects of the therapies you have selected?
3. **Assessment**
   a. Did the patient in this case study initially or subsequently demonstrate any evidence of the *clinical manifestations* of chronic bronchitis? What were they?
   b. Did the patient in this case study initially demonstrate any evidence of the *pathophysiologic alterations* associated with chronic bronchitis? What did it include?
   c. What *specific clinical manifestations* did this patient initially demonstrate that helped you determine the *severity* of his condition?
4. **Application**
   a. Oxygen therapy (was/was not) indicated because _____
   b. Monitoring (was/was not) indicated because _____
   c. Bronchial hygiene therapy (was/was not) indicated because _____
   d. Postural drainage (PD) and percussion (were/were not) indicated because

   _____
   e. Pulmonary rehabilitation (should/should not) be used in the comprehensive care of this patient because _____
5. **Evaluation**
   a. What are the expected outcomes of each aspect of therapy you have selected?
   b. How will you *monitor* patient response?
   c. What are the upper limits on the *intensity* and *frequency* of administration of each therapy?
   d. What are the *advantages* and *disadvantages* of each treatment modality?
   e. What if the patient improves?
   f. What if he does not improve?
6. **Boundary Awareness**
   a. How would you know that *this* patient is not improving or getting worse?
   b. When should you ask a supervisor for help?
   c. When should you call the patient's physician?
   d. How would you recognize actual or impending ventilatory failure in this patient?
   e. What adverse effects are there in the treatments you have selected?

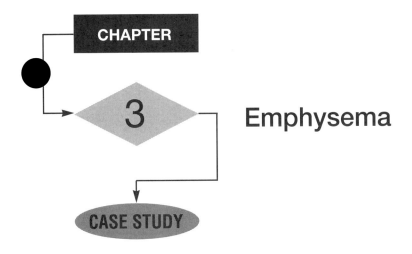

Emphysema

ADMITTING HISTORY

This 62-year-old man had a long history of cough and shortness of breath and multiple hospitalizations. He was admitted because of severe, worsening dyspnea. He had lived and worked in Pittsburgh, Pennsylvania, for 35 years as a foundry worker in a steel manufacturing plant. His wife had died 10 years earlier. After his wife's death, he had lived alone for 9 years and had managed his daily activities with progressive difficulty.

Two years before this admission he had been forced to retire early because of declining health. His doctor at that time told him he had chronic emphysema. For the past year he has lived with his brother's family in Chicago. During the interview the patient's brother indicated that his brother might "have the flu again." Although he had a 35 pack-year history of smoking unfiltered cigarettes, the patient had stopped smoking at the time of his forced retirement.

His last hospitalization was 9 weeks before this admission. At that time he was hospitalized for 2 days for cough, muscle aches and pains, fever, and respiratory distress. He underwent a complete pulmonary function study and received bronchial hygiene therapy, oxygen therapy, and instruction in at-home breathing exercises.

Also at this time it was noted the patient's expiratory flow rate measurements had declined significantly since his pulmonary function tests a year earlier. In fact, his forced expiratory volume in 1 second (FEV_1) had declined from 70% of predicted to 45% of predicted in the past year. At discharge 9 weeks before this admission and on 1.5 L/min O_2 by nasal cannula, the patient's arterial blood gas values were pH 7.37, Pa_{CO_2} 67 mm Hg, HCO_3^- 36 mmol/L, and Pa_{O_2} 63 mm Hg. He had received influenza vaccine 6 months earlier and pneumococcal vaccine 2 years earlier.

At the time of discharge 9 weeks earlier he was pursed-lip breathing and using his accessory muscles of inspiration at rest. He demonstrated no spontaneous cough or sputum production. His bronchodilator therapy had been discontinued at the discharge 1 year ago because it had been found to be "ineffective" during his pulmonary function study. He had been strongly encouraged to perform his pulmonary rehabilitation exercises on a daily basis. A weekly exercise flow chart had been provided for him at discharge by the respiratory care department.

PHYSICAL EXAMINATION

In the emergency room the patient was febrile, cyanotic, and in obvious respiratory distress. He appeared malnourished. He was 180 cm (6 ft tall) and weighed 66 kg (146 lb). He was cyanotic, and his skin was cool and clammy to the touch. The patient said, "I'm so short of breath."

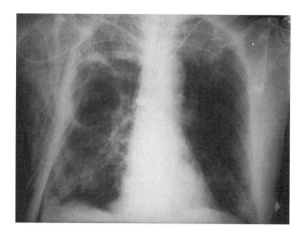

Fig. 3-1

His vital signs were blood pressure 155/110, heart rate 95 bpm, respiratory rate 25/min, and oral temperature 38.3° C (101° F). He was using his accessory muscles of inspiration and pursed-lip breathing. An enlarged anteroposterior diameter of the chest could easily be seen. Percussion revealed that he had low-lying hemidiaphragms. Expiration was prolonged, and his breath sounds were diminished. However, crackles could be heard over the right lower lobe.

A chest x-ray film showed pulmonary hyperexpansion, severe apical pleural scarring, a large bleb in the right middle lobe, and a right lower lobe infiltrate consistent with pneumonia (Fig. 3-1). Upon instruction, the patient's forced cough was weak and productive of a small amount of yellow sputum. On 2 L/min O_2 by nasal cannula, his arterial blood gases were pH 7.59, Pa_{CO_2} 40 mm Hg, HCO_3^- 37 mmol/L, and Pa_{O_2} 38 mm Hg. The physician ordered a pulmonary consult and stated that she did not want to commit the patient to a ventilator if possible.

RESPONSE 1

On the basis of the above information, write your SOAP in the following space.

S _____

_____

O _____

_____

_____

_____

_____

_____

_____

A _____

_____

_____

_____
_____
_____
_____
_____
_____

P _____
_____
_____
_____
_____
_____

6 HOURS LATER

At this time the patient stated that his chest was feeling tighter and that he was more short of breath. His vital signs were blood pressure 160/115, heart rate 97 bpm, respiratory rate 15/min and shallow, and oral temperature 37.8° C (100° F). He was no longer using his accessory muscles of inspiration or pursed-lip breathing. His breath sounds were diminished bilaterally, and crackles could no longer be heard over the right lower lobe. Dull percussion notes were elicited over the right lower lobe. His arterial blood gas values were pH 7.28, $Paco_2$ 82 mm Hg, HCO_3^- 36 mmol/L, and Pao_2 41 mm Hg. His hemoglobin oxygen saturation measured by pulse oximetry (Spo_2) was 68%.

RESPONSE 2

On the basis of the above information, write your SOAP in the following space.

S _____

O _____
_____
_____
_____
_____
_____
_____
_____

A _____
_____
_____

_____

_____

_____

_____

P _____

_____

_____

_____

_____

_____

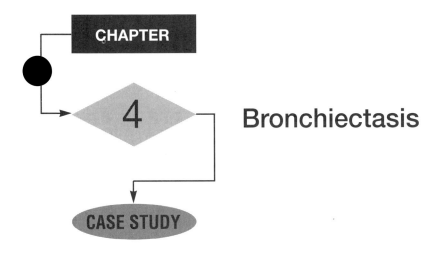

4 Bronchiectasis

CASE STUDY

ADMITTING HISTORY

This 56-year-old black woman was well known to the medical staff because of frequent episodes of upper respiratory infections. The patient worked 40 or more hours per week as a file clerk at a local health department and was known as a hard worker. Despite what she described as her "chronic cold," she rarely missed a day of work, although she frequently needed to request permission to leave work early because of doctor appointments. Fortunately, her immediate supervisor was a compassionate person and understood the patient's health problem and frequent requests to leave work early.

The patient's hospital chart showed that her respiratory problems began when she was in her early teens. During that period, frequent upper respiratory tract infections and an annoying cough were her only symptoms. It was also reported that she was a smoker of about 1 pack of cigarettes per day during her teen years. Over the years she had quit and restarted smoking many times. For the past several years she had treated herself with aerosolized bronchodilators and kept a humidifier running in her room most of the time. She frequently was given antibiotics in an alternating cycle. Her husband often administered chest physical therapy at home; she found this helpful for acute flare-ups (cough and increased sputum production).

The patient stated that she had not smoked for 3 months. Over the last 6 months, however, she stated that she had lost weight and had lost her generally "good spirits." She further stated that her cough was almost continuous, with production of copious amounts of foul smelling, purulent sputum. She denied hemoptysis. She also indicated that her coworkers had become concerned about her condition and had recommended that she seek immediate medical attention.

PHYSICAL EXAMINATION (Time: 0930)

The patient presented as a well-nourished female complaining of severe, nearly constant shortness of breath, a frequent, strong cough, and purulent sputum production. She appeared cyanotic, and her fingers and toes demonstrated mild clubbing. She was pursed-lip breathing and using her accessory muscles of inspiration. During each coughing episode she produced large amounts of foul smelling, yellow-green sputum.

Her vital signs were blood pressure of 185/90, heart rate 110 bpm, respiratory rate 30/min, and oral temperature 37.9° C (100.2° F). Palpation of the chest and percussion of the lungs revealed no remarkable abnormalities. On auscultation, bilateral rhonchi and persistent crackles over the lung bases could be heard.

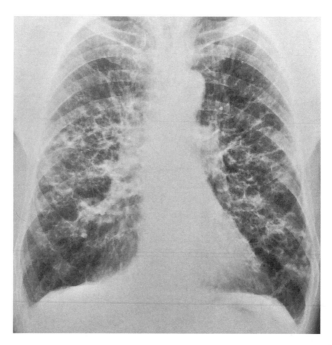

Fig. 4-1

Examination of her chart revealed mild-to-moderate airway obstruction on her last pulmonary function tests (PFT) performed 2 years ago. Her history also showed these baseline arterial blood gas values (ABGs) (on 2 L/min O_2): pH 7.38, Pa_{CO_2} 55 mm Hg, HCO_3^- 33 mmol/L, Pa_{O_2} 68 mm Hg. On this day, her bedside peak expiratory flow rate (PEFR) was 325 L/min, and her arterial blood gases on 3 L/min O_2 by nasal cannula were pH 7.52, Pa_{CO_2} 35 mm Hg, HCO_3^- 27 mmol/L, and Pa_{O_2} 53 mm Hg. Her chest x-ray film revealed cystic bronchiectasis, alveolar hyperinflation, and generalized increased bronchovascular markings (Fig. 4-1). The physician called for a respiratory care consult and stated that he did not want to commit the patient to a mechanical ventilator.

RESPONSE 1

On the basis of the above information, write your SOAP in the following space.

S _____

_____

O _____

_____

_____

_____

_____

_____

_____

_____

A _____

_____

_____

_____

_____

_____

_____

_____

P _____

_____

_____

_____

_____

_____

2 DAYS AFTER ADMISSION

The respiratory care practitioner assigned to the patient noted that she continued to experience respiratory distress. When questioned, the patient indicated that she had felt short of breath for several hours. She was cyanotic, pursed-lip breathing, and using her accessory muscles of respiration. She continued to cough frequently and produced large amounts of foul smelling, blood-streaked, yellow-green sputum. The sputum culture revealed *Streptococcus pneumoniae* and *Pseudomonas aeruginosa*.

Her vital signs were blood pressure 188/95, heart rate 118 bpm, respiratory rate 34/min, and oral temperature 37° C (98.6° F). Palpation and percussion of the chest were not remarkable. On auscultation, bilateral rhonchi and crackles could be heard over the lung bases. Bronchial breath sounds could be heard over the right lower lung base. Her oxygen saturation measured by pulse oximetry (Sp_{O_2}) was 93%. Her arterial blood gas values were pH 7.54, Pa_{CO_2} 30 mm Hg, HCO_3^- 28 mmol/L, and Pa_{O_2} 57 mm Hg. A current chest x-ray film revealed an opacity in the right lower lobe that was consistent with atelectasis or acute pneumonia.

RESPONSE 2

On the basis of the above information, write your SOAP in the following space.

S _____

_____

O _____

_____

_____

A _____

_____

_____

_____

_____

_____

P _____

_____

_____

_____

_____

4 DAYS AFTER ADMISSION

During an assessment and treatment session the patient stated she was breathing much better. Although she was still pale, there was no remarkable cyanosis, pursed-lip breathing, or use of accessory muscles of respiration. When asked to produce a strong cough, she did so and produced a moderate amount of thin, clear secretions. Her vital signs were blood pressure 135/85, heart rate 80 bpm, respiratory rate 14/min, and normal temperature. Mild rhonchi and crackles were still auscultated over the bases of both lung fields. Her Spo_2 was 94%, and her arterial blood gas values were pH 7.48, $Paco_2$ 49 mm Hg, HCO_3^- 38 mmol/L, and Pao_2 66 mm Hg. A current chest x-ray film showed no opacity in the right lower lobe.

RESPONSE 3

On the basis of the above information, write your SOAP in the following space.

S _____

O _____

_____

_____

_____

A

P

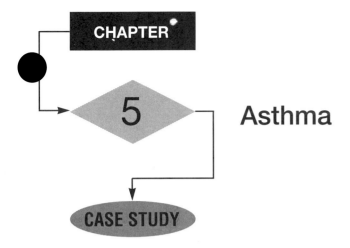

CHAPTER

5   Asthma

CASE STUDY

ADMITTING HISTORY

This 10-year-old girl was well known to the respiratory care protocol team. Over the past 8 years she had been hospitalized for severe asthma three or four times a year. She averaged 2- to 3-day hospital stays per admission. Over the past 4 years she had required mechanical ventilation three separate times. Because of her excessive absenteeism from school, the patient was held back in the second grade. At the time of this admission the patient was in the fourth grade.

About 2 years ago the patient's mother lost her job as a teller at a local bank because of the many days she needed to take off from work to take her daughter to the doctor. For the past 15 months the mother had been able to work only part time as a check-out clerk at a local grocery store. This turn of events further compromised an already extensive and growing medical bill.

The last time the patient was on a ventilator was about 2 years ago. After that hospitalization her mother—a single parent—quit smoking, a habit she had had for about 20 years, and the family cat was given away. In addition, the patient's mobile home and heating system were cleaned thoroughly, and several portable air-conditioning units were installed. For the past 6 months the patient had been on an albuterol inhaler four times a day and as needed, a beclomethasone inhaler four times a day, and theophylline twice daily. Her mother had been instructed in how to monitor her daughter's peak expiratory flow rate (PEFR) on a regular basis. The patient's personal best PEFR was about 290 L/min.

During a recent doctor's appointment, skin tests were found to be positive for ragweed and grasses. She was begun on a program of hyposensitization. Despite these efforts the patient still had a number of bad asthmatic episodes. Two episodes required hospitalization. Mechanical ventilation was not required in either case.

The patient was last hospitalized 6 weeks earlier. Her PEFR on admission was 175 L/min, and she had severe hypoxemia. At that time she received aerosolized terbutaline almost continuously for 3 hours and oxygen therapy per protocol. The physician on duty treated her aggressively with intravenous aminophylline and steroids. The patient progressively improved. Her arterial blood gas values returned to normal within 6 hours of her admission. She was discharged the next afternoon. Fortunately, because the asthma episode occurred over a weekend, no school days were missed.

About 6 hours before this admission the patient went to bed at 9 PM with no respiratory complaints, although she had been achy and tired for about 1 week. At about 1:30 AM she awoke short of breath. After alerting her mother, she took two puffs of her albuterol inhaler. Her mother then measured her daughter's PEFR and noted that it was 235 L/min. Hoping that this asthma episode would soon subside, she had her daughter take another puff of her inhaler. She then encouraged her daughter to try and go back to sleep.

Within 45 minutes, however, the patient's condition had not improved and, in fact, was getting progressively worse. Her PEFR at this time was 210 L/min. Again the mother had her daughter take two puffs of her albuterol inhaler. Ten minutes later the mother again had her daughter forcefully exhale into her peak flow meter. Her PEFR was 170 L/min. At this point she put her daughter, still in her pajamas, into the car and drove to the hospital emergency room.

PHYSICAL EXAMINATION (Time: 0315)

On admission to the emergency department the patient had extreme shortness of breath. She was sitting up Indian style on the hospital gurney, with her hands and arms in front of her anchored to her knees in a tripod position. She was using her accessory muscles of inspiration and pursed-lip breathing and was crying, anxious in appearance, and cyanotic. She stated, "I feel horrible, and my chest is tight." She frequently demonstrated a strong productive cough. Her sputum was moderate in quantity and thick and white.

Her PEFR was 150 L/min. Her heart rate was 190 bpm; her blood pressure was 110/85, and she had a respiratory rate of 28/min. Her temperature was normal. On auscultation, she had diminished breath sounds, wheezing, and rhonchi bilaterally. Her chest x-ray film showed severe air trapping with depressed hemidiaphragms and hyperlucency of the lungs (Fig. 5-1). Her hemoglobin oxygen saturation measured by pulse oximetry (Sp_{O_2}) on 2 L/min O_2 by cannula was 77%, and her arterial blood gases were pH 7.45, Pa_{CO_2} 28 mm Hg, HCO_3^- 19 mmol/L, and Pa_{O_2} 40 mm Hg. The physician had the patient transferred to the pediatric intensive care unit (ICU). A respiratory care consult was requested. On the patient's chart the physician had written, "Respiratory care—please assess and treat as aggressively as our protocol boundaries permit. I want to keep this patient off the ventilator if possible."

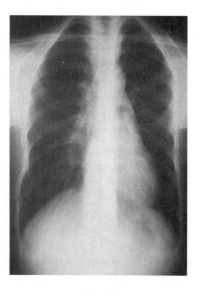

Fig. 5-1

RESPONSE 1

On the basis of the above information, write your SOAP in the following space.

S _____

_____

O _____

_____

_____

_____

_____

_____

_____

A _____

_____

_____

_____

_____

_____

_____

P _____

_____

_____

_____

_____

_____

TIME: 0530 (Same Day)

Since her admission, neither the patient nor her mother had been able to sleep. The patient was in a high Fowler's position with her arms fixed to the side bed rails. She was using her accessory muscles of inspiration and pursed-lip breathing and was cyanotic. She had a frequent, strong cough that produced a moderate amount of thick, white secretions during each coughing episode. Her chest still appeared to be hyperinflated. She stated, "I'm sorry. I'm wheezing too much, and I can't go to sleep."

Her PEFR at this time was 175 L/min. Her heart rate was 180 bpm, blood pressure 105/82, and respiratory rate 24/min. Hyperresonant percussion notes were produced bilaterally. On auscultation, she demonstrated prolonged expiration, diminished breath sounds, rhonchi, and wheezing bilaterally. No follow-up chest x-ray film had been taken. Her Sp_{O_2} was 95%, and her arterial blood gas values were pH 7.48, Pa_{CO_2} 34 mm Hg, HCO_3^- 24 mmol/L, and Pa_{O_2} 73 mm Hg.

RESPONSE 2

On the basis of the above information, write your SOAP in the following space.

S _____

_____

O _____

_____

_____

_____

_____

_____

_____

A _____

_____

_____

_____

_____

_____

_____

P _____

_____

_____

_____

_____

_____

TIME: 0745 (Same Day)

The day shift therapist assigned to the patient gathered this clinical data during her morning rounds: The patient stated that she felt like a weight was on her chest. She was using her accessory muscles of inspiration and pursed-lip breathing. Her skin was damp and cool, and she was cyanotic. No cough or sputum production was noted. Her PEFR was 145 L/min. Her vital signs were blood pressure 160/100, heart rate 185 bpm, and respiratory rate 13/min. Her breath sounds were diminished bilaterally, and no wheezes or rhonchi were heard during auscultation. Hyperresonant percussion notes were elicited bilaterally. Her Sp_{O_2} was 79%, and her arterial blood gas values were pH 7.27, Pa_{CO_2} 57 mm Hg, HCO_3^- 24 mmol/L, and Pa_{O_2} 51 mm Hg.

RESPONSE 3

On the basis of the above information, write your SOAP in the following space.

S _____

_____

O _____

_____

_____

_____

_____

_____

_____

A _____

_____

_____

_____

_____

_____

_____

P _____

_____

_____

_____

_____

_____

1. Basic Concept Formation
a. Are *children* affected with asthma?

b. Are *adults* affected with asthma?

c. Is the *cause* of asthma hyperreactivity of the airway to allergic substances?

d. Is the *treatment* of asthma *simple?* Is it always *successful?*

e. Are the main *clinical manifestations* of asthma cough and sputum production? If not, what are the common *clinical manifestations* of asthma?

f. Are patients or caregivers of patients with asthma allowed to *increase or decrease their treatment* on the basis of the clinical manifestations?

g. What class(es) of inhaled agents are commonly used as treatment by symptomatic asthmatics?

h. What is the *time course* of asthma? Over hours? Over days? Over the life of the patient?

2. Data Base Formation
a. What is your *vision* of the pathology of bronchial asthma?

b. What are the *various types* of asthma?

c. What *pathophysiologic mechanisms* are activated as a result of the typical anatomic alterations?

d. What portion(s) of the *airway model* (Fig. 1-3) is/are abnormal in asthma?

e. What are the *goals of therapy* for asthmatic patients? What constitutes *"good control"* of asthma?

f. Which *standard modalities* should help achieve these goals?

g. List the modalities' typical therapies ordered, expected outcomes, and monitors.

3. Assessment
a. Did this patient initially or subsequently demonstrate any evidence of the *clinical manifestations* of bronchial asthma? If so, what were they?

b. Did this patient initially demonstrate any evidence of the *pathophysiologic alterations* associated with bronchial asthma?

c. What *specific clinical manifestations* of asthma did this patient initially demonstrate that helped you determine the *severity* of her condition?

4. Application
a. Oxygen therapy (was/was not) indicated in this patient because _____.

b. Monitoring (was/was not) indicated because _____.

c. Bronchial hygiene therapy (was/was not) indicated because _____.

d. Bronchodilator or antiinflammatory aerosol therapy (was/was not) indicated because _____.

e. Hyperinflation therapy (was/was not) indicated because _____.

f. Intubation *or* mechanical ventilation (was/was not) *initially* indicated because _____.

5. Evaluation
a. What are the expected outcomes of each aspect of therapy you have selected?

b. How can you *monitor* the patient's response?

c. What are the upper limits of the *intensity or frequency* of administration of each modality?

d. What are the *advantages* of each treatment modality?

e. What if the patient improves?

f. What if she does not?

6. Boundary Awareness
a. How can you tell that *this* patient is not improving or getting worse?

b. Can the patient or her parent or caregiver be of any help should she worsen?

c. When should you ask a supervisor for help?

d. When should you contact the patient's physician?

e. How would you recognize actual or impending ventilatory failure in this patient?

f. What *dangers* are there in the treatment(s) you have selected in her case?

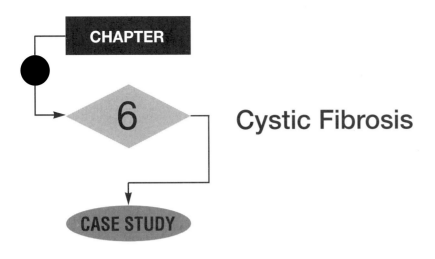

CHAPTER

6 Cystic Fibrosis

CASE STUDY

ADMITTING HISTORY

This 27-year-old man had a long history of respiratory problems due to cystic fibrosis. Even though his medical records were not complete, he reported that his parents had told him that he had had several episodes of pneumonia during his early years. The patient was an adopted child and therefore did not know his family history. The patient's parents were actively involved in his general care, which entailed the home care suggestions or therapeutic procedures presented by the pulmonary rehabilitation team. The patient took supplemental multivitamins and timed-release pancreatic enzymes on a regular basis as prescribed by his doctor.

During his teens he had fewer respiratory symptoms and was able to live a pretty normal life. It was during that time that he took up waterskiing and became proficient in the slalom event. He was known to most of his associates as a "wonder." Although he qualified for disability because of his continual shortness of breath, he was able to do various small jobs, which always related to waterskiing. He was well known throughout the waterskiing circuit as an excellent chief judge at national and regional tournaments. He was a certified driver for jump trick and slalom events and recently had become involved in selling waterski tournament ropes and handles, which provided him with a small additional income.

In the past 3 years his cough had become more persistent and increasingly productive with about a cupful of sputum noted daily. Over the same period he had noted intermittent hemoptysis and had become short of breath when climbing stairs. Even though the patient had a normal appetite, he had lost a great deal of weight over the past 2 years. He denied any recent changes in bowel habits despite his weight loss but had noticed a tendency to pass rather pale stools. Much to the chagrin of his doctor, he started smoking 3 years ago and smoked about 10 cigarettes a day, his reason being that the cigarettes helped him cough up the sputum.

PHYSICAL EXAMINATION

On examination the patient appeared pale, cyanotic, and thin. He had a barrel chest and was using his accessory muscles of respiration. There was clubbing of the fingers. He demonstrated a frequent, productive cough. His sputum was sweet smelling, thick, and yellow-green. His neck veins were distended, and he showed mild-to-moderate peripheral edema. He stated that he had not been this short of breath in a long time.

He had a respiratory rate of 28/min, a blood pressure of 142/90, and a heart rate of 108 bpm. He was afebrile. Palpation of the chest was not remarkable. Expiration was prolonged. Hyperresonant notes were elicited bilaterally during per-

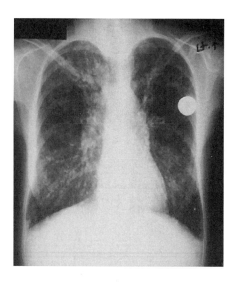

Fig. 6-1

cussion. Auscultation revealed diminished breath sounds and heart sounds. Crackles and rhonchi were heard throughout both lung fields.

His chart showed that during his last medical check-up (about 10 months before this admission) a pulmonary function study was conducted. Results showed the patient had moderate-to-severe airway obstruction. No blood gases were analyzed.

His chest x-ray film on this admission revealed hyperlucent lung fields, depressed hemidiaphragms, and right ventricular enlargement (Fig. 6-1). His arterial blood gas values while he was on 1.5 L/min oxygen by nasal cannula were pH 7.51, Pa_{CO_2} 58 mm Hg, HCO_3^- 43 mmol/L, and Pa_{O_2} 66 mm Hg. His hemoglobin oxygen saturation measured by pulse oximetry (Sp_{O_2}) was 94%.

RESPONSE 1

On the basis of the above clinical information, write your SOAP in the following space.

S _____

_____

O _____

_____

_____

_____

_____

_____

_____

_____

A _____

_____

_____

_____

P _____

48 HOURS AFTER ADMISSION

The respiratory therapist from the respiratory care consult service noted that the patient was again in respiratory distress. The patient stated that he could not get enough air to sleep even 10 minutes. He was cyanotic and using his accessory muscles of respiration. His vital signs were respiratory rate 32/min, blood pressure 147/95, heart rate 117 bpm, and temperature 37° C (98.6° F).

He coughed frequently, and even though his cough was weak, he produced large amounts of thick, green sputum. Hyperresonant notes were produced during percussion over both lung fields. On auscultation, breath sounds and heart sounds were diminished. Crackles, rhonchi, and wheezing were heard throughout both lung fields. No recent chest x-ray film was available. A sputum culture confirmed the presence of *Pseudomonas aeruginosa.* His Spo_2 was 92%. His arterial blood gas values were pH 7.55, $Paco_2$ 54 mm Hg, HCO_3^- 45 mmol/L, and Pao_2 57 mm Hg.

RESPONSE 2

On the basis of the above clinical information, write your SOAP in the following space.

S _____

O _____

A _____

_____
_____
_____
_____
_____

P _____
_____
_____
_____
_____
_____

64 HOURS AFTER ADMISSION

At this time the respiratory care practitioner noted the patient was in obvious respiratory distress. The patient indicated he could not get into a position to breathe comfortably. He appeared cyanotic and was pursed-lip breathing and using his accessory muscles of respiration. His vital signs were respiratory rate 22/min; blood pressure 145/90; and heart rate 120 bpm. Palpation was normal, and bilateral hyperresonant percussion notes were elicited. Auscultation revealed crackles, rhonchi, and wheezing bilaterally. No recent chest x-ray film was available. His Spo_2 was 65%, and his arterial blood gases were pH 7.33, $Paco_2$ 79 mm Hg, HCO_3^- 41 mmol/L, and Pao_2 37 mm Hg.

RESPONSE 3

On the basis of the above clinical information, write your SOAP in the following space.

S _____
_____

O _____
_____
_____
_____
_____
_____
_____
_____

A _____
_____
_____
_____

P

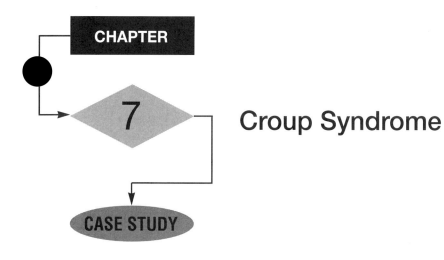

7 Croup Syndrome

ADMITTING HISTORY

Three days before Christmas this 3-year-old boy was a typical, healthy child. He was energetic and curious, and his attention span was short. He generally played well with other children, and at his day care center he was well liked and considered a happy child by the staff. On this day, however, he often became frustrated and angry, and at one point a staff member had to stop a fight between the patient and a little girl. The staff member noted that the boy's face appeared flushed and felt warm to the touch. Because the flu was going around, it was thought that the patient could be coming down with it. At this point the patient's mother was called.

At home the mother checked her son's temperature and found it to be normal. Because he felt warm, however, she gave him some liquid acetaminophen (Tylenol). For lunch the patient ate about three bites of a peanut butter sandwich, drank about half a glass of juice, and ate some grapes. Although his mother wanted him to take a nap, he insisted that he was not tired. The patient then began to play with his father's Lionel train underneath the Christmas tree. Ten minutes later the patient was asleep while the train was still running around the tree. His mother then placed him in his bed.

Although the patient slept through the night, he was lethargic the next morning and frequently complained to his mother that he did not feel good. Even though the patient's temperature was 37° C (98.6° F), the mother gave him some more liquid acetaminophen. For breakfast he ate a few bites of cereal and had some juice. He then wrapped himself in a blanket in front of the television set. He coughed occasionally during this time. By noon the mother noticed that her son's cough was more frequent and had a barking quality. She also noted that her son's voice sounded hoarse. By late afternoon the patient's condition had progressively worsened, and he told his mother he was having trouble breathing. Becoming worried, the mother carried him to the car and drove him to the hospital emergency room.

PHYSICAL EXAMINATION

On inspection the patient was sitting up and in obvious respiratory distress. He demonstrated a frequent brassy cough, and inspiratory stridor was clearly present. He was flushed, very anxious, gasping for air, and crying quietly. His apical pulse was 160 bpm, his respiratory rate 58/min, and his blood pressure 110/70. His temperature was normal. Chest examination showed obvious intercostal and su-praclavicular retractions. Palpation and percussion were not remarkable. Normal, but diminished breath sounds were auscultated. His oxygen saturation measured by pulse oximetry (Sp_{O_2}) while he was on an oxygen mask was 88%. The attending physician ordered a chest x-ray film.

On the basis of the above clinical information, write your SOAP in the following space.

S _____

_____

O _____

_____

_____

_____

_____

_____

_____

A _____

_____

_____

_____

_____

_____

_____

_____

P _____

_____

_____

_____

_____

_____

1 HOUR LATER

Despite the treatment given, the patient still appeared to be in respiratory distress. He had intercostal and supraclavicular retractions. His inspiratory stridor showed no change, and his cough was still frequent and brassy sounding. In a hoarse voice, he said he wanted to go home. His vital signs were blood pressure 146/88, apical pulse 155 bpm, respiratory rate 63/min, and temperature normal. His chest x-ray film showed a subglottic haziness (Fig. 7-1). Fig. 7-2 is a close-up of the neck region of Fig. 7-1. Breath sounds were normal but diminished. His SpO_2 was 90%.

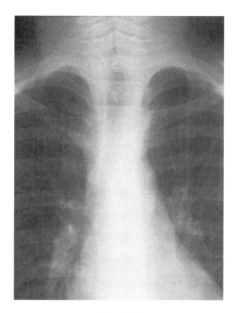

Fig. 7-1

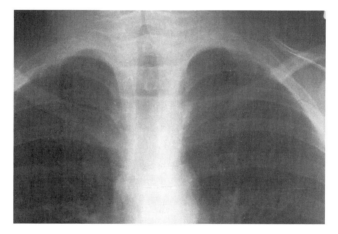

Fig. 7-2

RESPONSE 2

On the basis of the above clinical information, write your SOAP in the following space.

S _____

_____

O _____

_____

_____

_____

_____

_____

A _____

_____

_____

_____

_____

_____

_____

_____

P _____

_____

_____

_____

_____

_____

CHRISTMAS EVE

At 0130 the physician called the respiratory care consult service to evaluate the patient's respiratory status and make any recommendations they could regarding the patient's discharge status. The respiratory care practitioner found the patient sitting up in his bed coloring. The patient nodded when asked if he felt better. Inspiratory stridor no longer could be heard, and intercostal or supraclavicular retractions no longer could be seen. His apical pulse was 89 bpm; his respiratory rate was 15/min, and his blood pressure was 125/80. Breath sounds were normal. His Sp_{O_2} was 97%.

RESPONSE 3

On the basis of the above clinical information, write your SOAP in the following space.

S _____

_____

O _____

_____

_____

_____

_____

_____

_____

A

P

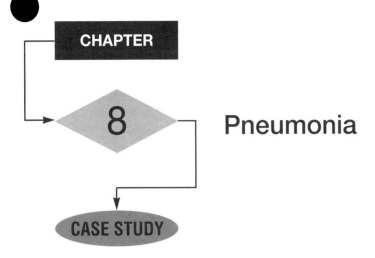

CHAPTER

8 Pneumonia

CASE STUDY

ADMITTING HISTORY

This 79-year-old man was admitted to the hospital because of cough, fever, and a right lower lobe infiltrate. He was born in Detroit and worked as a truck driver for a dry cleaning chemicals company for 51 years. He was always a hard worker and an active member of Teamsters Local 299. As a truck driver, it was not uncommon for him to be on the road 3 to 4 days at a time.

He never married, and after his sister died when he was 55 years old, he no longer had any living relatives. He started smoking when he was 14 years old and averaged about two packs of cigarettes a day. When he was not working, he consumed alcohol on a regular basis. Despite his smoking and drinking habits, he retired in good health at 65 years of age.

The patient was last admitted to the hospital 2 years ago for an acute inferior myocardial infarction. He was treated with medications and recovered quite well. He stopped smoking at that time but continued to consume alcohol on a regular basis. He reported that he generally consumed about four to six bottles of beer each night at a local bar with some of his old retired "buddies." After his myocardial infarction, he continued to manage his daily affairs without difficulty. He exercised regularly by working in his yard each day, and he power-walked every other day at the mall.

Four days before this admission the patient reported that he had "flulike" symptoms. He had chills, a mild fever, and a hacking, nonproductive cough. Although he was not feeling well, he continued to work in his yard and power-walk at the mall. He also socialized and consumed beer with his friends each night. The evening before this admission his friends noted that he was progressively getting worse and encouraged him to see a doctor. Thinking he would get better soon, he stated that if he did not feel better in a week or so he would go see his doctor. The next day, however, the patient was very short of breath, his cough was more frequent, and he had a temperature of 38.3° C (101° F). At that point he drove himself to the hospital.

PHYSICAL EXAMINATION

On inspection the patient was a well-nourished man in obvious respiratory distress on 2 L/min O_2 by nasal cannula. He was monitored by pulse oximetry. The patient

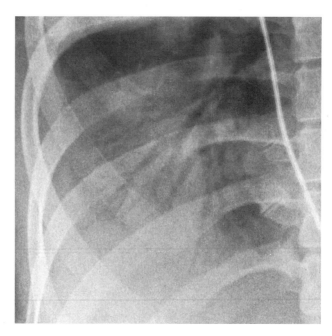

Fig. 8-1

stated that he was very short of breath. He had a blood pressure of 165/90, heart rate of 120 bpm, respiratory rate of 33/min, and an oral temperature of 39.5° C (103° F). He demonstrated a frequent, strong cough. His cough was "hacky" and productive of a small amount of white and yellow sputum. His skin appeared pale and damp. When the patient repeated the phrase ninety-nine, there was increased tactile and vocal fremitus over the right lower lung posteriorly. Dull percussion notes and bronchial breath sounds were noted over the right lower lung regions posteriorly. His oxygen saturation measured by pulse oximetry (Spo_2) was 92%, and his arterial blood gases were pH 7.56, $Paco_2$ 24 mm Hg, HCO_3^- 22 mmol/L, and Pao_2 56 mm Hg. His chest x-ray film demonstrated a right lower lobe infiltrate consistent with pneumonia, air bronchograms, and alveolar consolidation (Fig. 8-1). His WBC count was 21,000/mm³.

RESPONSE 1

On the basis of the above information, write your SOAP in the following space.

S _____

_____

O _____

_____

_____

_____

_____

A _____

P _____

6 HOURS LATER

The therapist doing assessment rounds gathered the following clinical information: The patient stated, "My doctor is too young. I feel worse than when I came in here." He had a blood pressure of 140/70, a heart rate of 125 bpm, a respiratory rate of 35/min and shallow, and a temperature of 38.9° C (102° F). He demonstrated a strong, "barking" cough, and during each major coughing episode he produced a small amount of blood-streaked sputum.

His skin was cyanotic. Over his right lower and middle lobes and his left lower lobe, he demonstrated increased tactile and vocal fremitus, dull percussion notes, bronchial breath sounds, and crackles. His Spo_2 was 91%. His arterial blood gas values were pH 7.55, $Paco_2$ 26 mm Hg, HCO_3^- 24 mmol/L, and Pao_2 53 mm Hg.

RESPONSE 2

On the basis of the above information, write your SOAP in the following space.

S _____

O _____

A _____

_____

_____

_____

_____

_____

_____

P _____

_____

_____

_____

_____

THE NEXT DAY

The respiratory therapist assigned to evaluate the patient gathered this clinical information: The patient stated that he slept most of the night and was breathing easier. The patient's blood pressure was 135/85; his heart rate was 90 bpm; his respiratory rate was 19/min; and he had an oral temperature of 37.3° C (99° F). He had a strong, nonproductive cough.

His morning chest x-ray film and report indicated partial resolution of the pneumonic process but persistent consolidation or atelectasis in the right lower and middle lobes and left lower lobe. In these lung areas the tactile and vocal fremitus had increased, and dull percussion notes and bronchial breath sounds were heard. His Spo_2 was 97%. His arterial blood gases were pH 7.44, $Paco_2$ 35 mm Hg, HCO_3^- 24 mmol/L, and Pao_2 163 mm Hg.

RESPONSE 3

On the basis of the above information, write your SOAP in the following space.

S _____

_____

O _____

_____

_____

A

P

➥ KEY POINT Questions   **For Pneumonia (DRG 89)**

---

1. **Basic Concept Formation**
   a. Is pneumonia an *allergic* disorder? Is it usually caused by an *infectious* agent? Is it sometimes *contagious?*
   b. Are cough and fever common *clinical manifestations* of pneumonia?
   c. What class of drugs is almost always used in the *treatment* of pneumonia?
   d. Can pneumonia be *fatal?*

2. **Data Base Formation**
   a. What is your *vision of the pathology* of acute pneumonia?
   b. What are the *common causes* of pneumonia? Are they different in different segments of the population?
   c. What *pathophysiologic mechanisms* are activated as a result of the typical anatomic alterations?
   d. How is *severe* community-acquired pneumonia (CAP) *defined?*
   e. What are current criteria for *hospitalization* of patients with CAP?
   f. What are the *goals of therapy* for hospitalized patients with pneumonia?
   g. What *standard TDPs* would most likely help achieve these goals?
   h. What are the common *complications* of pneumonia?

3. **Assessment**
   a. Is the patient in this case study initially or subsequently demonstrating any classic *clinical manifestations* of pneumonia? If so, what are they?
   b. Did this patient demonstrate any evidence of the *pathophysiologic abnormalities* commonly associated with acute pneumonia?
   c. What specific *clinical manifestations* of pneumonia helped you decide on the severity of his condition?

4. **Application**
   a. Sputum sample/induction (was/was not) indicated in this patient because
   _____.
   b. Oxygen therapy (was/was not) indicated because _____.
   c. Bronchial hygiene therapy (was/was not) indicated because _____.
   d. Bronchodilator therapy (was/was not) indicated because _____.
   e. Hyperexpansion therapy (was/was not) indicated because _____.

5. **Evaluation**
   a. What are the expected outcomes of each therapeutic modality you have selected?
   b. How can you *monitor* the patient's response to therapy?
   c. What are the upper limits of the intensity of therapy you have started on this patient?
   d. What would you do if the patient's *oxygenation worsened* or if CO_2 *retention and respiratory acidemia* occurred?

6. **Boundary Awareness**
   a. How can you tell that *this* patient is not improving or getting worse?
   b. In this case, should you have called for the supervisor after the first assessment?
   c. When should you call the physician in this case?
   d. How (did/would) you recognize impending ventilatory failure in this patient?

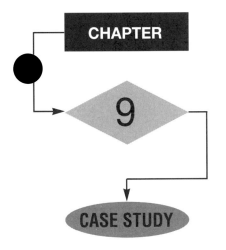

9

Acquired Immunodeficiency Syndrome (AIDS)

CASE STUDY

ADMITTING HISTORY

This 26-year-old white man entered the emergency room complaining of a sore throat and persistent cough. He stated that his ability to swallow had progressively worsened over the last 2 weeks. At this time he indicated that the pain was so severe that he was unable to eat solid food and that he had begun to find it difficult to swallow fluids.

Obtaining a history was difficult. The patient's answers were often vague, and he rarely looked the nurse in the eyes as he spoke. The patient denied any major medical problems. The nurse learned that about 8 months before this admission the patient had the flu for about a week and received treatment for a rash on his back. It was shortly after this period that the patient recalled first noticing the irritating cough, which had persisted to the present time.

The patient also had a history of a low hemoglobin, for which he took iron tablets. He admitted to previous intravenous drug use but stated that he had been drug free for the past 2 months. He confirmed he had no family physician, and when he did become ill, he would go to various emergency rooms and clinics in the area.

The patient said that he occasionally had symptoms of upper respiratory tract infection with nasal congestion and a loose cough productive of clear, white sputum. He also said that he had chills and night sweats, sometimes so severe that he had to change his clothes and bed linens. Finally, he noted that he had become increasingly tired over the past several weeks.

PHYSICAL EXAMINATION

The patient appeared as a pale, malnourished white man sitting upright with his legs hanging over the side of the gurney and his hands and arms to his side, bracing himself on the side of the gurney. He had mild facial acne, a slight rash on his anterior chest and neck, and two herpes-like blisters on his lower lip. He stated that his throat was "killing him" and that his cough was "driving him nuts!" During the physical examination he frequently demonstrated a strong, nonproductive cough.

His vital signs were blood pressure 137/90, heart rate 95 bpm, respiratory rate 20/min, and temperature 37° C (98.6° F). Lymph nodes in his neck were noted to be swollen. Dull percussion notes were produced over his lung bases, and bronchial breath sounds were auscultated over the same areas. His chest x-ray film showed infiltrates in both lower lung fields consistent with pneumonia (Fig. 9-1). His arterial blood gas values on room air were pH 7.47, $Paco_2$ 33 mm Hg, HCO_3^- 23 mmol/L, and Pao_2 76 mm Hg. The physician called for a respiratory consult and requested an induced sputum sample for a Gram stain and sputum culture.

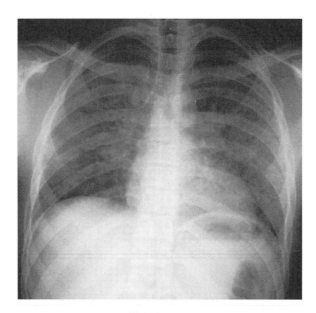

Fig. 9-1

On the basis of the above information, write your SOAP in the following space.

S _____

_____

O _____

_____

_____

_____

_____

_____

_____

_____

A _____

_____

_____

_____

_____

_____

_____

P _____

_____

_____

_____

3 DAYS LATER

The respiratory care practitioner found the patient lying in bed and short of breath. He stated, "I'm not breathing very well. I'm getting worse." He coughed every few minutes. The cough was strong and nonproductive. His vital signs were blood pressure 185/100, heart rate 125 bpm, respiratory rate 31/min, and temperature 37° C (98.6° F). Over the right middle and lower lobes and the left lower lobe, dull percussion notes and bronchial breath sounds were found. No recent chest x-ray film was available. His oxygen saturation measured by pulse oximetry (Sp_{O_2}) was 92%, and his arterial blood gas values were pH 7.54, Pa_{CO_2} 27 mm Hg, HCO_3^- 22 mmol/L, and Pa_{O_2} 54 mm Hg. A sputum culture produced normal respiratory flora.

RESPONSE 2

On the basis of the above information, write your SOAP in the following space.

S _____

_____

O _____

_____

_____

_____

_____

_____

_____

A _____

_____

_____

_____

_____

_____

P _____

_____

_____

_____

THE NEXT DAY

Concerned with the patient's deteriorating respiratory status, the nurse working with the patient called the respiratory care consult service and requested an update. Upon entering the room, the respiratory therapist observed the patient to be dyspneic and in obvious respiratory distress. Although the patient was awake, he generally kept his eyes closed and just turned his head from side to side when the therapist asked how he was feeling. No cough was noted at this time. His vital signs were blood pressure 170/85, heart rate 145 mm Hg, respiratory rate 30/min and shallow, and rectal temperature 40° C (104° F).

His morning chest x-ray film showed greater infiltration and air bronchograms throughout the right middle and lower lung lobes and the left lower lung lobe. A second laboratory screening test showed the patient's blood was positive for anti-HIV antibodies. A Western blot assay was ordered. Spo_2 was 77%, and his arterial blood gas values were pH 7.28, $Paco_2$ 61 mm Hg, HCO_3^- 27 mmol/L, and Pao_2 47 mm Hg.

RESPONSE 3

On the basis of the above information, write your SOAP in the following space.

S _____

_____

O _____

_____

_____

_____

_____

_____

_____

_____

A _____

_____

_____

_____

_____

_____

_____

_____

P _____

_____

_____

_____

_____

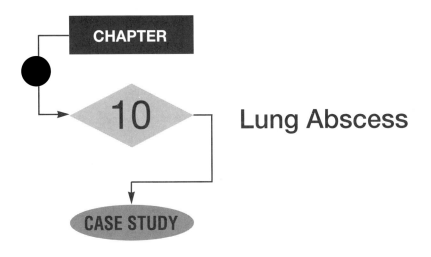

CHAPTER

10 Lung Abscess

CASE STUDY

ADMITTING HISTORY

This 36-year-old Spanish American woman had been "homeless" for the past 15 years and had lived "on the streets" most of the time. When the weather was very cold, she generally entered a downtown shelter. She had a long history of alcohol abuse, although she had had no alcohol during the preceding year. She was a heavy smoker and had been known to smoke up to three or four packs of cigarettes a day. Despite her rough living conditions, her personal hygiene, in general, appeared good.

Over the past 3 years the patient had been seen by a physician who volunteered at the downtown clinic on a weekly basis. The entire medical staff was familiar with her condition, as in the past they had treated her for her alcohol-related problems, hypothermia during one especially cold winter, numerous bouts of pneumonia, and for various scrapes, cuts, and broken bones caused by frequent falls. Before visiting the health clinic this time, however, the patient had seemed better and even indicated that she had a better outlook on life. On this day, though, the physician was concerned to see the patient back at the clinic and looking poorly.

PHYSICAL EXAMINATION

On physical examination the patient appeared as a thin, undernourished female with a disheveled appearance. She was found sitting in the upright position and leaning forward on the bedside table. The patient said, "I spit all the time." She was cyanotic, and her teeth and mouth were in especially poor condition. She had a weak-to-moderate, frequent cough productive of foul smelling purulent sputum. After each coughing episode she wiped her mouth and nose with her sleeve.

Even though she did not appear intoxicated, her speech was nearly unintelligible, and she was confused. Her skin was dirty, and several bruises could be seen on her arms and legs. The patient's street partner gave a history that the patient had been losing weight, appeared tired all the time, and had felt excessively warm for the preceding week.

Her vital signs were blood pressure 145/75, heart rate 110 bpm, respiratory rate 33/min, and temperature 39.3° C (102.8° F). Auscultation revealed crackles and rhonchi over the right middle and lower lung lobes. Normal vesicular breath sounds were heard over the left lung. Tactile and vocal fremitus were noted over the right lung. Her arterial blood gas values on 2 L/min oxygen by nasal cannula were pH 7.49, $Paco_2$ 30 mm Hg, HCO_3^- 22 mmol/L, and Pao_2 63 mm Hg. Her chest x-ray film revealed a partially fluid-filled, 10 cm cavity formation in the right upper lobe and increased opacity in both the middle and right lower lobes (Fig. 10-1).

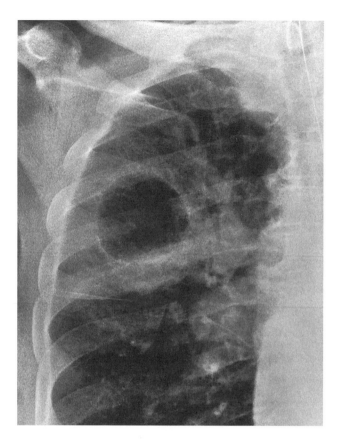

Fig. 10-1

RESPONSE 1

On the basis of the above information, write your SOAP in the following space.

S _____

_____

O _____

_____

_____

_____

_____

_____

_____

_____

A _____

_____

_____

_____

_____
_____
_____
_____

P _____
_____
_____
_____
_____
_____

24 HOURS LATER

During morning rounds the respiratory care practitioner working on the consult team noted that the patient still had a frequent, weak cough, and she continued to expectorate thick, purulent sputum. The patient stated, however, that she did not feel as short of breath as the day before. Overall, she appeared better and more alert, but she was still cyanotic. Compared to the day before, her speech was more intelligible.

Her vital signs were blood pressure 135/80, heart rate 98 bpm, respiratory rate 20/min, and temperature 37.9° C (100.2° F) (she was currently on aspirin). Over the right middle and lower lobes, tactile and vocal fremitus were documented, and crackles and rhonchi were heard on auscultation. Her arterial blood gas values were pH 7.48, $Paco_2$ 34 mm Hg, HCO_3^- 23 mmol/L, and Pao_2 81 mm Hg. Her hemoglobin oxygen saturation measured by pulse oximetry (Spo_2) was 96%.

RESPONSE 2

On the basis of the above information, write your SOAP in the following space.

S _____

O _____
_____
_____
_____
_____
_____
_____

A _____
_____
_____

_____
_____
_____
_____
_____

P _____
_____
_____
_____
_____

3 DAYS LATER

At this time the patient stated, "You doctors cured my damn cough!" The patient's skin no longer appeared cyanotic, and no spontaneous cough was noted. When asked to force a cough, the patient produced a strong cough, but no sputum production was noted. Her vital signs were blood pressure 127/82, heart rate 86 bpm, respiratory rate 16/min, and normal temperature.

No tactile or vocal fremitus could be detected over the right middle and lower lobes. Crackles, however, could still be auscultated over the right lower lobe. Her arterial blood gas values were pH 7.43, $Paco_2$ 36 mm Hg, HCO_3^- 24 mmol/L, and Pao_2 163 mm Hg. Her Spo_2 was 97%. Although the morning chest x-ray film still revealed the partially fluid-filled abscess, the infiltrate in the right lower lung lobe was improved. Some infiltrate was still seen around the abscess in the right middle lobe.

RESPONSE 3

On the basis of the above information, write your SOAP in the following space.

S _____
_____

O _____
_____
_____
_____
_____
_____
_____

A _____
_____

P

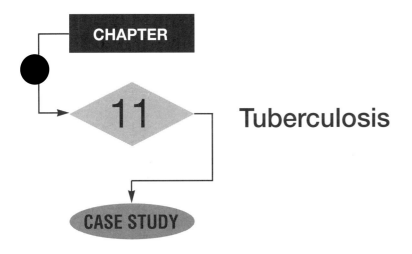

CHAPTER

11 Tuberculosis

CASE STUDY

ADMITTING HISTORY

This 58-year-old white man was well known and liked by the staff at the Samaritan Shelter for the Homeless. The social workers at the shelter had spent a great deal of time and resources in working with the patient through a number of areas, including his alcohol addiction. Their records showed that they had not seen the patient for about 6 months. When they had last seen him, he was not drinking, had just secured a job as a janitor at a large department store, and was making enough money to eat and pay the rent on a small apartment.

The staff was saddened when he came to the shelter in search of some food and a bed. The patient appeared tired, dirty, and depressed. He smelled of alcohol. He stated that he had quit his job about 3 months before this admission because his boss was "a jerk." He also confirmed that he had been out on the streets again because of his inability to pay the rent. Although he chain smoked as he talked to the staff, he frequently complained about his "smoker's cough."

Two days after he arrived at the shelter the patient started having episodes of coughing that were more severe than usual. On several occasions the coughing spells lasted for more than 2 hours. Hemoptysis often occurred during these periods. When the staff at the shelter noted that the patient had expectorated about a pint of fresh blood, it was decided to transfer him to the local charity hospital. Although the patient was initially quite resistant, he finally agreed to go to the hospital.

PHYSICAL EXAMINATION

In the emergency room the patient appeared anxious, chronically and acutely malnourished, weak, and in obvious respiratory distress. His nail beds were cyanotic, and his fingers were yellow from nicotine stains. The patient stated that he had smoked approximately 30 cigarettes a day for 35 years. He had a frequent, strong cough, producing moderate amounts of yellow sputum mixed with small amounts of fresh blood. He stated that his cough had been getting worse, and he thought that he probably had "a cold." He also indicated that he could not seem to get his breath.

The patient denied any respiratory problems before this admission. However, he also stated that coughing up blood was no "big deal," since he had done it a couple of times before. Although the patient denied having used alcohol for months, the staff from the shelter documented the smell of alcohol when he came to them. It could be seen that the patient had obviously fallen in the recent past. He had several large bruises on his forehead, right shoulder and arm, and over his right anterior axillary chest region between the sixth and ninth ribs.

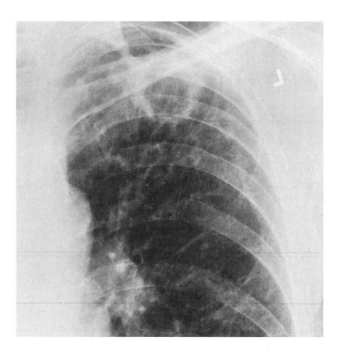

Fig. 11-1

The patient's vital signs were blood pressure 170/95, heart rate 110 bpm, respiratory rate 26/min, and temperature 38.3° C (101° F). Although palpation of the chest was negative, dull percussion notes and increased tactile and vocal fremitus were noted over the lung bases. Bronchial breath sounds were heard over the right and left lung bases. Crackles and rhonchi were noted over the right upper lobe. A pleural friction rub was also auscultated over the right lower lobe between the fifth and sixth ribs in the anterior axillary line.

A chest x-ray film revealed an increased opacity consistent with pneumonia in the left lower lobe and right middle and upper lobes. A 5 cm cavity could easily be seen in the left upper lobe (Fig. 11-1). The patient had a hemoglobin level of 17 g/dl and a WBC of 14,000/mm^3. While the patient was in the emergency room, the nurse administered a Mantoux tuberculin skin test. The patient's arterial blood gas values on room air were pH 7.53, Pa_{CO_2} 51 mm Hg, HCO_3^- 41 mmol/L, and Pa_{O_2} 50 mm Hg. His carboxyhemoglobin level was 8.5%, and his hemoglobin oxygen saturation measured by pulse oximetry (Sp_{O_2}) was 88%.

RESPONSE 1

On the basis of the above information, write your SOAP in the following space.

S _____

_____

O _____

_____

●

A _____

P _____

●

●

4 DAYS AFTER ADMISSION

In reviewing the patient's chart the respiratory care practitioner noted that the patient had a positive tuberculin reaction. An acid-fast stain and sputum culture had been ordered. It was also noted that the patient had undergone fiberoptic bronchoscopy. During this procedure, both old and fresh blood were found throughout the tracheobronchial tree. Secretions obtained from the large airways were negative for malignant cells.

A complete pulmonary function study (PFT) indicated a moderate-to-severe restrictive disorder. The morning chest x-ray film showed an improvement in the aeration of the lung bases as compared to the admission radiograph. The patient's cyanosis and respiratory distress appeared better. His cough was still frequent and productive. The amount of sputum, however, was not as great as on admission. Although the sputum was opaque, it was no longer yellow, and no blood could be seen. The patient stated that his cough was a lot better.

His vital signs were blood pressure 143/90, heart rate 92 bpm, respiratory rate 18/min, and temperature 37.4° C (99.3° F). Dull percussion notes and bronchial breath sounds were noted over the lung bases. Rhonchi could still be heard over the right middle lobe, although they were not so pronounced as on admission. The pleural friction rub was no longer present. The patient's arterial blood gas values were pH 7.48, $Paco_2$ 60 mm Hg, HCO_3^- 42 mmol/L, Pao_2 61 mm Hg. His Spo_2 was 91%.

RESPONSE 2

On the basis of the above information, write your SOAP in the following space.

S _____

_____

O _____

_____

_____

_____

_____

_____

_____

_____

A _____

_____

_____

_____

_____

_____

_____

_____

P _____

_____

_____

_____

_____

_____

7 DAYS AFTER ADMISSION

As part of the discharge team on this day the respiratory care practitioner reviewed the patient's chart and noted that the patient's morning chest x-ray film had significantly improved. The parenchymal densities present in the lung bases on admission were much improved. The large cavity in the upper left lung lobe, however, was still clearly visible. While in the hospital, the patient had been started on daily dosages of isoniazid and rifampin (Rifadin). Arrangements had been made with the staff at Samaritan Shelter to dispense the prescribed drugs and to monitor the patient's compliance in taking them.

On observation, the patient still appeared moderately pale and cyanotic, but he no longer appeared to be in respiratory distress. In addition, he no longer demonstrated a spontaneous, uncontrolled cough. The patient stated that he was ready to run a marathon. When asked to cough, the patient generated a strong, nonproductive cough. His vital signs were blood pressure 135/85, heart rate 80 bpm, respiratory rate 10/min, and oral temperature 37° C (98.6° F). Palpation and percussion were essentially negative. Normal vesicular breath sounds were heard over the lower lung fields. On a 1 L/min O_2 nasal cannula the patient's arterial blood gas values were pH 7.42, Pa_{CO_2} 72 mm Hg, HCO_3^- 45 mmol/L, and Pa_{O_2} 78 mm Hg. His Sp_{O_2} was 94%. Sputum smears showed acid-fast bacilli (presumed *Mycobacterium tuberculosis*). Routine sputum cultures were negative; acid-fast cultures were pending.

RESPONSE 3

On the basis of the above information, write your SOAP in the following space.

S _____

O _____

A _____

P _____

12

Fungal Diseases of the Lungs

CASE STUDY

ADMITTING HISTORY

This 56-year-old cattle driver was admitted to the arthritis clinic of a small hospital just outside of Phoenix because of joint pain. The patient stated that the tenderness in his joints prevented him from riding his horse for any extended period. He was born on a cattle ranch in New Mexico and had spent most of his adult life working as a cattle driver in Arizona, New Mexico, and Colorado. He had always considered himself an "outdoors" kind of man. He loved the range, the wide open spaces, the clear air, and the beauty of the desert.

In his early twenties he traveled to the East Coast to go to college. While there, he became withdrawn, depressed, and felt confined. After 1 year he dropped out of college and returned to New Mexico. Shortly after being back home, his symptoms of depression disappeared. He was working on a large cattle ranch, had made several new friends, and was content with the fact that he belonged on the open range. He never married or settled down in one place he could call home. He often said that the great outdoors was his home. He never owned an automobile. In fact, he often said that the only things of real value he owned were a roan quarter horse and a saddle.

The hospital had no past medical record on the patient. The patient claimed, however, that although he was rarely ill, he had gone to see a doctor about a year ago while in Colorado for severe "cold" symptoms, which included fever, cough, chest pain, headaches, and a general tired feeling. He was a nonsmoker, although he did chew tobacco for a short time in his teens. The patient verified that he consumed alcohol on a regular basis on Friday and Saturday nights. On an average, the patient estimated that he consumed between six and ten beers per outing and sometimes more. Despite the patient's somewhat rugged living conditions and alcohol consumption, he was not overweight and was in reasonably good physical condition.

PHYSICAL EXAMINATION

The patient presented as a well-developed, well-nourished white man in moderate respiratory distress. He complained of soreness and stiffness of all his joints. He also stated that he thought he had a "bad cold" and that he was short of breath.

The patient's knees and ankle joints were swollen and tender to the touch. Although his skin appeared weathered and tan, his lips and nail beds were cyanotic. He demonstrated a frequent cough productive of a moderate amount of thick, yellow sputum. Although the patient's cough was strong, he had a difficult time raising sputum during each coughing episode. His vital signs were blood pressure 160/90, heart rate 93 bpm, respiratory rate 18/min and oral temperature 37.8° C (100° F).

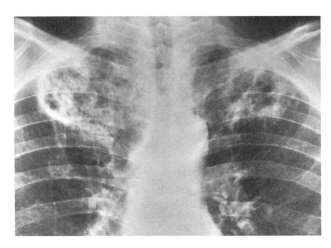

Fig. 12-1

Palpation revealed a few erythematous lesions on his anterior chest. The patient was not aware of these. There was also a walnut-size erythematous lesion on the patient's left cheek. Percussion of the chest was not remarkable. Auscultation revealed bilateral crackles and rhonchi in the lung bases.

The patient's chest x-ray film showed scattered infiltrates consistent with fibrosis and calcification and multiple spherical nodules throughout both lungs. In the upper lobes of both lungs, two to three small, 1- to 3-cm, cavities could be seen (Fig. 12-1). On room air the patient's arterial blood gas values were pH 7.51, $Paco_2$ 29 mm Hg, HCO_3^- 22 mmol/L, and Pao_2 64 mm Hg. Concerned about the patient's respiratory status, the physician requested a respiratory care consult.

RESPONSE 1

On the basis of the above information, write your SOAP in the following space.

S _____

_____

O _____

_____

_____

_____

_____

_____

_____

_____

A _____

_____

_____

_____

●
_____
_____
_____
_____
_____

P _____
_____
_____
_____
_____
_____

5 DAYS AFTER ADMISSION

The respiratory care practitioner (RCP) working with the patient at this time gathered the following clinical information from the patient's chart: Based on microscopy of the patient's sputum and a spherulin skin test, the diagnosis of coccidioidomycosis was now written in the patient's chart. The patient had been receiving amphotericin B intravenously for 2 days. A complete pulmonary function study revealed a moderate-to-severe restrictive disorder.

●
When the RCP entered the patient's room, the patient was sitting up in bed, appearing cyanotic, short of breath, and fatigued. He stated that he was getting real tired of people in white outfits coming in and out of his room, day and night, with needles, pills, and bills. He further stated that he still could not get a good breath of air. In fact, he said it was more difficult for him to breathe today than it had been on the day he entered the hospital.

The patient still had a frequent, strong cough productive of moderate amounts of thick, opaque sputum. His vital signs were blood pressure 165/95, heart rate 97 bpm, respiratory rate 24/min, and normal temperature. Auscultation revealed persistent bilateral crackles and rhonchi in the lung bases. A current chest x-ray film was not available. His hemoglobin oxygen saturation measured on pulse oximetry (Sp_{O_2}) was 88%. His arterial blood gas values were pH 7.54, Pa_{CO_2} 27 mm Hg, HCO_3^- 21 mmol/L, and Pa_{O_2} 55 mm Hg.

RESPONSE 2

On the basis of the above information, write your SOAP in the following space.

S _____

O _____
_____
_____
●
_____
_____

A _____

_____

_____

_____

_____

_____

_____

_____

P _____

_____

_____

_____

_____

_____

10 DAYS AFTER ADMISSION

On this day the respiratory therapist found the patient walking up and down the corridor talking to various staff members and patients. The patient appeared to be in no respiratory distress. The patient stated that he was breathing much better and that he was ready to ride his horse a long distance in any direction away from the hospital.

No spontaneous cough was noted. When asked to generate a cough, the patient produced a strong, nonproductive cough. His vital signs were blood pressure 135/88, heart rate 80 bpm, respiratory rate 14/min, and normal temperature. Auscultation revealed bilateral crackles in the lung bases. A recent chest x-ray film was not available. His pulse oximetry showed an Spo_2 of 91%. His arterial blood gas values were pH 7.44, $Paco_2$ 34 mm Hg, HCO_3^- 23 mmol/L, and Pao_2 71 mm Hg.

RESPONSE 3

On the basis of the above information, write your SOAP in the following space.

S _____

_____

O _____

_____

_____

_____

A

P

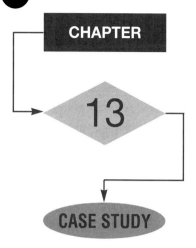

CHAPTER

13

Pulmonary Edema

CASE STUDY

ADMITTING HISTORY

This 68-year-old hypertensive man arrived in the emergency department via ambulance at 0645. The patient's wife stated that her husband was doing well until the evening before admission, when he complained of being tired and short of breath. She also noted that he had a sudden onset of dry, nonproductive cough. Thinking that he was getting a "touch of the flu," she made her husband some hot soup, gave him two aspirins and a tablespoon of Robitussin, and made him go to bed at about 8:30 PM. About 4:30 AM she stated that she awoke to find her husband sitting up in bed, gasping for air. Alarmed, she called 911.

The patient's previous history showed him to be in fairly good health since his retirement as a plumber 2 years ago. He had smoked about one pack of cigarettes a day for the past 40 years. For the past 2 years he and his wife had actively devoted most of their time to gardening and travel. They were planning a cross-country trailer trip to Alaska. About 1 year ago the patient had a physical examination in preparation for this trip. At that time the patient's physician placed him on digoxin and furosemide (Lasix) for atrial fibrillation and mild congestive heart failure. The patient quit smoking.

Upon the patient's arrival at the treatment room the emergency room nurse immediately placed him in a high Fowler's position. The respiratory therapist started oxygen at 2 L/min by nasal cannula. His wife appeared anxious. She was sobbing and walking back and forth and stating repeatedly, "Bill takes a heart pill and a water pill, and he follows a low salt diet—just like the doctor told him to do."

PHYSICAL EXAMINATION (Time 0700)

Upon inspection the patient was in obvious respiratory distress. The patient stated, however, "I don't think I'm having a serious problem." He further stated, "My wife and I are only 2 days away from our dream trip to Alaska. We've been planning this trip for 8 years! I can't believe this! . . . It is just 2 days before we are supposed to leave, and here I am on this emergency room gurney!"

His vital signs were blood pressure 175/130, heart rate 145 bpm and irregular, and respiratory rate 22 breaths per minute. His throat was reddened. On 2 L/min O_2, his lips were blue, his neck veins were distended, he appeared very anxious, and he was coughing frequently and producing small amounts of frothy, pink secretions. His abdomen was distended, and there was pitting edema to midcalf.

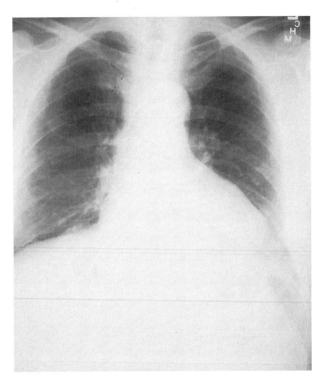

Fig. 13-1

Palpation of his chest was unremarkable. Dull percussion notes were elicited over the lower lung regions bilaterally. Auscultation revealed inspiratory crackles and expiratory wheezing over the left and right lower lung regions.

His arterial blood gases on 2 L/min O_2 by nasal cannula were pH 7.56, Pa_{CO_2} 28 mm Hg, HCO_3^- 20 mmol/L, Pa_{O_2} 61 mm Hg. According to the radiologist's report, his chest x-ray film showed dense, fluffy opacities over the lower lung areas bilaterally. The x-ray report also noted that the patient's heart was moderately enlarged, suggesting left ventricular hypertrophy (Fig. 13-1).

The emergency room physician started the patient on intravenous digitalis, dobutamine, and furosemide. The physician ordered another chest x-ray film and asked the respiratory care consult service to see the patient. He specifically requested that respiratory care monitor the patient closely over the next several hours.

RESPONSE 1

On the basis of the above information, write your SOAP in the following space.

S _____

_____

O _____

_____

_____

_____

_____

A _____

P _____

TIME: 1100

The repeat bedside chest x-ray film showed no remarkable improvement. The patient stated, "I still don't feel great." The patient's vital signs were blood pressure 160/125, heart rate 105 bpm and regular rhythm, and respiratory rate 20 breaths per minute. The color of his lips had improved slightly, but there appeared to be no improvement in the patient's distended neck veins. The nurse noted that the patient's urine output over the past 2 hours had been 650 ml. The patient still coughed frequently; however, there was no frothy, pink sputum noted at this time. Auscultation continued to reveal inspiratory crackles and expiratory wheezing over the lower lung lobes bilaterally. His pulse oximetry showed an Spo_2 of 84%. This observation was followed by an arterial blood gas study that revealed pH 7.54, $Paco_2$ 25 mm Hg, HCO_3^- 18 mmol/L, and Pao_2 51 mm Hg.

RESPONSE 2

On the basis of the above information, write your SOAP in the following space.

S _____

O _____

A _____

_____

_____

_____

_____

_____

_____

P _____

_____

_____

_____

_____

TIME: 1630

The patient stated that he was breathing better. The patient's vital signs were blood pressure 140/115, heart rate 95 bpm and regular, and respiratory rate 16 breaths per minute. His lips and fingertips were no longer blue. The nursing chart showed that the patient's urine output over the past 2 hours had been 850 ml. The patient appeared relaxed, and there was no longer any significant venous distension. Upon request, the patient produced a strong, nonproductive cough. Auscultation revealed bilateral crackles over the lower lung lobes. His pulse oximetry showed an SpO_2 of 97%, and repeated arterial blood gases were pH 7.44, $PaCO_2$ 36 mm Hg, HCO_3^- 24 mmol/L, and PaO_2 190 mm Hg.

RESPONSE 3

On the basis of the above information, write your SOAP in the following space.

S _____

O _____

_____

_____

_____

_____

_____

A _____

_____

_____

_____

_____

_____

_____

P _____

_____

_____

_____

_____

_____

◦→ KEY POINT QUESTIONS   *For Pulmonary Edema (DRG 87)*

1. **Basic Concept Formation**
   a. Is *heart failure* associated with dyspnea?
   b. What happens to *pulmonary venous pressure* if the *left heart fails*?
   c. What is the meaning of *edema*?
   d. Are the *risk factors* for heart disease and lung disease similar?

2. **Data Base Formation**
   a. What is your *vision of the pathology* of acute pulmonary edema?
   b. What *pathophysiologic mechanisms* are activated as a result of these anatomic alterations?
   c. What *clinical manifestations* might be observed if these pathophysiologic mechanisms are activated?
   d. What *other signs and symptoms* might be seen in cases of pulmonary edema?
   e. What should be the *goals of therapy* in such patients?
   f. Which *standard TDPs* might achieve these goals?
   g. List the *outcomes* and potential *adverse effects* of each protocol you have selected and describe how you would *monitor* their beneficial and adverse effects.

3. **Assessment**
   a. Did the patient in this case study have any *risk factors* for cardiac disease and congestive heart failure?
   b. Did this patient initially or subsequently demonstrate any of the *clinical manifestations* of acute pulmonary edema? What were they?
   c. Did the patient in this case study initially demonstrate any evidence of the *pathophysiologic alterations* typically associated with pulmonary edema?
   d. What *specific clinical manifestations* did this patient demonstrate that helped you decide on the *severity* of his condition?

4. **Application**
   a. Oxygen therapy (was/was not) indicated because _____.
   b. Monitoring (was/was not) indicated because _____.
   c. Bronchial hygiene therapy (was/was not) indicated because _____.
   d. Bronchodilator therapy (was/was not) indicated because _____.
   e. Hyperinflation therapy (was/was not) indicated in this case because
      _____.
   f. Mechanical ventilation (was/was not) indicated in this case because
      _____.

5. **Evaluation**
   a. What are the expected *results* of each modality or protocol that you have selected?
   b. How will you *monitor* the patient's response to these therapies?
   c. How can you increase or decrease the *intensity* or *frequency* of each modality as needed?
   d. What are the *advantages and disadvantages* of each treatment modality?
   e. How will you *reduce therapy* in this case *if the patient improves*?

6. **Boundary Awareness**
   a. How would you know that this patient is not improving or actually getting worse?
   b. When should you ask a supervisor for help?
   c. When should you call the patient's physician?
   d. How would you recognize actual or impending respiratory failure in this patient?
   e. What dangers are there in the treatments you have selected?

14 Pulmonary Embolism

ADMITTING HISTORY

This 32-year-old motorcycle enthusiast who smoked one pack of cigarettes per day fell asleep while riding his bike with a group of Harley "hogs" to the annual Sturgis Rally in North Dakota. Although there was extensive damage to his motorcycle, the patient did remarkably well and was conscious when the ambulance arrived. Before he was transported to the local hospital, he was worked on in the field; splints and an immobilizer were applied. His injuries were thought to include a fractured pelvis, left tibia, and left knee.

Enroute to the hospital a partial rebreathing oxygen mask was placed over the patient's face. An intravenous infusion was started with 5% glucose solution. The patient was alert and able to answer questions. The patient's vital signs were blood pressure 150/90, heart rate 105 bpm, and respiratory rate 20/min. Various small lacerations and scrapes on the patient's face and left shoulder were attended to. Each time the patient was moved slightly or when the ambulance suddenly bounced or turned sharply as it moved over the highway, the patient frequently complained of abdominal and bilateral chest pain. The emergency medical technician (EMT) crew all felt that his helmet and his youth saved his life.

In the emergency room a laboratory technician drew the patient's blood; several x-ray films were taken with a portable machine, and the patient's pain was treated with morphine. Within an hour the patient was taken to surgery to have the broken bones in his left leg repaired. Four hours later he was transferred to the intensive care unit (ICU) with his left leg in a cast. Thrombosis and embolism prophylaxis had been started with low-dose heparin. Busy with another surgery, the physician ordered a respiratory care consult on the patient.

PHYSICAL EXAMINATION

The respiratory therapist found the patient lying in bed with his left leg suspended about 25 cm (10 in) above the bed surface. He had a partial rebreathing oxygen mask on his face and was alert. His wife and two young boys around 10 years of age who were wearing black motorcycle jackets were at the patient's bedside. The patient stated he was feeling much better and that his breathing was okay.

His vital signs were blood pressure 115/75, heart rate 75 bpm, and respiratory rate 11/min. He was afebrile. His skin color was good. No remarkable breathing problems were noted. Palpation revealed mild tenderness over the patient's left shoulder and left anterior chest area. Percussion was not remarkable, and auscultation revealed normal vesicular breath sounds. The chest x-ray film taken earlier that morning in the emergency room was normal. His arterial blood gas values on a partial rebreathing mask were pH 7.40, Pa_{CO_2} 41 mm Hg, HCO_3^- 24 mmol/L, and Pa_{O_2} 504 mm Hg. His hemoglobin oxygen saturation measured by pulse oximetry (Sp_{O_2}) was 97%.

RESPONSE 1

On the basis of the above information, write your SOAP in the following space.

S _____

_____

O _____

_____

_____

_____

_____

_____

_____

A _____

_____

_____

_____

_____

_____

_____

_____

P _____

_____

_____

_____

_____

_____

3 DAYS AFTER ADMISSION

The patient's general course of recovery was uneventful until the third day, when the nurses noted swelling of the patient's left calf when giving him a bath. A Doppler study revealed a left tibial deep vein thrombosis. The physician was informed. Anticoagulant therapy was started. Five hours later the patient became short of breath and agitated. A spontaneous cough was noted, productive of a small amount of blood-tinged sputum. A pulmonary artery catheter was inserted. Concerned, the nurse called the physician and respiratory care.

When the respiratory care practitioner walked into the patient's room, the patient appeared cyanotic, was very short of breath, and stated that he felt awful. The patient further said that he had precordial chest pain, was lightheaded, and had a feeling of impending doom. The patient's vital signs were blood pressure 90/45, heart rate 125 bpm, respiratory rate 30/min, and oral temperature 37.2° C (99° F). Palpation and percussion of the chest were unremarkable. Auscultation revealed faint wheezing throughout both lung fields. A pleural friction rub could be heard anteriorly over the right middle lobe.

The patient demonstrated an electrocardiographic pattern that alternated between a normal sinus rhythm, sinus tachycardia, and atrial flutter. The patient's hemodynamic indices showed an increased central venous pressure (CVP), right atrial pressure (RAP), mean pulmonary artery pressure ($\overline{PA}$), right ventricular stroke work index (RVSWI), and pulmonary vascular resistance (PVR) and a decreased pulmonary capillary wedge pressure (PCWP), cardiac output (CO), stroke volume (SV), stroke volume index (SVI), and cardiac index (CI). The patient's chest x-ray film showed increased density in the right middle lobe consistent with atelectasis and consolidation. The patient's arterial blood gas values were pH 7.53, Pa_{CO_2} 26 mm Hg, HCO_3^- 21 mmol/L, and Pa_{O_2} 53 mm Hg. The patient's Sp_{O_2} was 89%. The physician started the patient on intravenous streptokinase, ordered a ventilation-perfusion scan, and requested that respiratory care see the patient again.

RESPONSE 2

On the basis of the above information, write your SOAP in the following space.

S _____

_____

O _____

_____

_____

_____

_____

_____

_____

A _____

_____

_____

_____

_____

_____

_____

P _____

_____

_____

_____

_____

_____

2 HOURS LATER

The patient's ventilation-perfusion scan showed no blood flow to the right middle lobe. The patient's eyes were closed, and he was no longer responsive to questions. The patient's skin appeared cyanotic, and his cough was productive of a small amount of blood-tinged sputum. The patient's vital signs were blood pressure 70/35, heart rate 160 bpm, and respiratory rate 25/min and shallow. Palpation of the chest was normal. Dull percussion notes were elicited over the right middle lung lobe. Wheezing was heard throughout both lung fields, and a pleural friction rub could be heard over the right middle lobe.

The patient demonstrated an electrocardiographic pattern that alternated between a normal sinus rhythm, sinus tachycardia, and atrial flutter. The patient's hemodynamic indices continued to show an increased CVP, RAP, $\overline{PA}$, RVSWI, and PVR and a decreased PCWP, CO, SV, SVI, and CI. The patient's arterial blood gas values were pH 7.25, Pa_{CO_2} 69 mm Hg, HCO_3^- 27 mmol/L, and Pa_{O_2} 37 mm Hg. The patient's Sp_{O_2} was 64%.

RESPONSE 3

On the basis of the above information, write your SOAP in the following space.

S _____

_____

O _____

_____

_____

_____

_____

_____

_____

A _____

_____

_____

_____

P

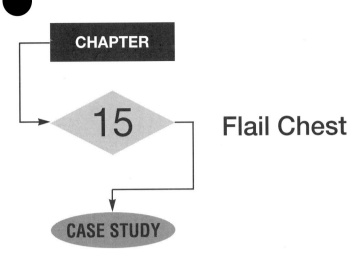

CHAPTER

15 — Flail Chest

CASE STUDY

ADMITTING HISTORY

This 22-year-old white man had a long history of alcohol abuse. While in middle school, he and his friends would steal their parents' beer and drink on a regular basis. By the time he was in his senior year in high school, he was drinking beer and Jack Daniel's whisky on almost a daily basis. He often became "mean" when he was drinking, and it was not unusual for him to get into fights. Although he was well built and was considered nice looking, he generally was not able to maintain a long-term relationship with the girls he dated in high school. At graduation, however, he was dating a girl whom he married 7 months later.

The marriage was a stormy one. His wife was well known to the social workers answering the hot-line phones at the local crisis center. On several occasions his wife called the police to their mobile home with reports of spousal abuse. One time he was waving a small handgun at her and accidently shot a hole through their kitchen wall. He would always apologize extensively to his wife after a major incident and promise, to no avail, to stop drinking.

Within 1 year of their marriage he lost his carpenter's job for missing too much work. Fifteen months after their wedding his wife had him served with a restraining order, filed for a divorce, and moved back in with her parents. He continued to drink heavily as he worked various minimum wage jobs for the next 2 years. Over the past 3 months he had been laid off for the winter season as an unskilled laborer by the local union. With his unemployment checks he spent most of his days and evenings in local bars drinking, playing cards, and shooting pool. Five weeks before this admission he lost his driver's license for a year for hitting—and totaling—a parked car while he was driving under the influence of alcohol.

On the day of this admission the patient started drinking heavily around 4 in the afternoon. By 11:30 PM he was at a local dance club and extremely intoxicated. He was using foul language, bumping into people, yelling out insults at the band, and constantly trying to start a fight with the other customers. The bouncer quickly ushered him off the premises.

The weather was bad on this night. It was cold, raining, sleeting, and dark as he walked and hitchhiked along a country road. He stumbled and staggered into the road as he walked along and yelled out profanities at the cars as they drove past. A witness later told the police that he appeared to dare the cars to hit him. Twenty minutes

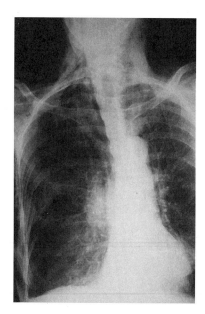

Fig. 15-1

after he was thrown out of the dance club, he was hit by a pickup truck. The ambulance crew found him 35 yards away from the road, lying in a corn field.

PHYSICAL EXAMINATION

When the patient was brought into the emergency room, he was unconscious but breathing on his own through a nonrebreathing mask. He had numerous scrapes and lacerations on his face, anterior chest, and legs. Both his upper and lower front teeth were broken off at the gum lines. Paradoxical movement could clearly be seen over most of his anterior chest. His skin was pale and cyanotic, and the smell of alcohol strongly radiated from his body. His blood alcohol level was 0.34%.

The patient's vital signs were blood pressure 165/92, heart rate 120 bpm, and respiratory rate 26/min and shallow. The patient's weight was about 86 kg (190 lb). Breath sounds were diminished bilaterally. A chest x-ray film showed extensive multiple double rib fractures of the right and left anterior and lateral ribs, between ribs 4 and 9. His sternum was fractured in three separate places. Increased densities, consistent with atelectasis, were seen throughout both lung fields in the chest x-ray film (Fig. 15-1). The patient's arterial blood gas values were pH 7.17, $Paco_2$ 82 mm Hg, HCO_3^- 27 mmol/L, and Pao_2 37 mm Hg. His hemoglobin oxygen saturation measured by pulse oximetry (Spo_2) was 59%.

RESPONSE 1

On the basis of the above information, write your SOAP in the following space.

S _____

_____

O _____

_____

_____

A _____

P _____

24 HOURS AFTER ADMISSION

The patient was still classified as in serious and unstable condition. He was on a mechanical ventilator in the controlled mode. A pulmonary artery catheter, central venous pressure catheter, and an arterial line were in place. Although the patient came in and out of consciousness, he was on a pancuronium (Pavulon) drip and was unable to move. No paradoxical movement of the chest could be detected.

His skin still appeared pale and cyanotic, and his neck veins were distended. The patient's vital signs were blood pressure 100/65, heart rate 145 mm Hg, and a controlled mechanical ventilation respiratory rate of 12 breaths per minute. No breath sounds could be heard over the right lung field. Diminished breath sounds were heard over the left lung lobes. Rhonchi and crackles could also be heard over the left lung fields.

A chest x-ray film taken earlier that morning by portable machine showed the left lung to be partially aerated with patches of atelectasis; the right lung was shown to be completely atelectatic. No pneumothorax was present. His hemodynamic status revealed an increased CVP, RAP, $\overline{PA}$, RVSWI, and PVR and a decreased PCWP, CO, SV, SVI, CI, LVSWI, and SVR.* His arterial blood gas values were pH 7.25, Pa_{CO_2} 65 mm Hg, HCO_3^- 25 mmol/L, and Pa_{O_2} 54 mm Hg. The patient's oxygenation status showed an increased $\dot{Q}s/\dot{Q}t$, $C(a-\bar{v})_{O_2}$, and O_2ER, and a decreased D_{O_2} and $S\bar{v}_{O_2}$.† His hemoglobin saturation measured by pulse oximetry (Sp_{O_2}) was 86%.

*CVP = central venous pressure, RAP = right atrial pressure, $\overline{PA}$ = mean pulmonary artery pressure, RVSWI = right ventricular stroke work index, PVR = pulmonary vascular resistance, PCWP = pulmonary capillary wedge pressure, CO = cardiac output, SV = stroke volume, SVI = stroke volume index, CI = cardiac index, LVSWI = left ventricular stroke work index, SVR = systemic vascular resistance.

†$\dot{Q}s/\dot{Q}\tau$ = cardiac output shunted/total cardiac output, $C(a-\bar{v})_{O_2}$ = arterial – mixed venous difference in oxygen concentration, O_2ER = oxygen extraction ratio, D_{O_2} = total oxygen delivery, $S\bar{v}_{O_2}$ = mixed venous oxygen saturation.

94 *Chest and Pleural Trauma*

RESPONSE 2

On the basis of the above information, write your SOAP in the following space.

S

O

A

P

72 HOURS AFTER ADMISSION

The patient's condition was classified as critical and unstable. His skin was cyanotic, and his neck veins were severely distended. His vital signs were blood pressure 80/32, heart rate 190 bpm, and a controlled mechanical ventilation respiratory rate of 14 breaths per minute. No breath sounds could be heard over the right lung field. Diminished breath sounds were heard over the left lung. Rhonchi and crackles could also be heard over the left lung fields. Large amounts of yellow sputum were being suctioned from the patient's endotracheal tube.

A chest x-ray film made by portable machine showed the left lung to be partially aerated, with patches of atelectasis that were more extensive than they had been 2 days before. The right lung was still shown to be airless. The radiologist also described early signs of adult repiratory distress syndrome (ARDS). No pneumothorax was present. The patient's electrocardiogram demonstrated periodic premature ventricular contractions.

All of the patient's hemodynamic values had worsened from earlier readings. His arterial blood gas values were pH 7.22, $Paco_2$ 71 mm Hg, HCO_3^- 24 mmol/L, and Pao_2 34 mm Hg. The patient's oxygenation status had progressively worsened from readings made 2 days earlier. His Spo_2 was 61%. The patient's family was called and the hospital priest was notified.

RESPONSE 3

On the basis of the above information, write your SOAP in the following space.

S _____

_____

O _____

_____

_____

_____

_____

_____

_____

A _____

_____

_____

_____

_____

_____

_____

P _____

_____

_____

_____

_____

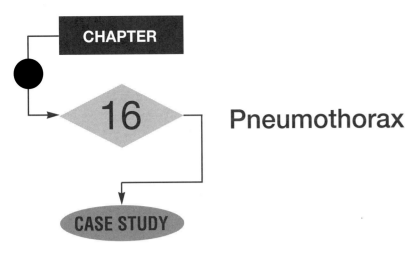

CHAPTER

16   Pneumothorax

CASE STUDY

ADMITTING HISTORY

This 64-year-old white man was well known to the respiratory care consult team. He had a long history of chronic bronchitis and emphysema. Although he had not been hospitalized in over 2 years, he had received extensive care 4 years earlier for a left lower lobe pneumonia that compromised his already severe chronic obstructive pulmonary disease (COPD). At that time he was placed on the ventilator for 17 days. His medical record showed that it was difficult to wean him from the ventilator for both pathophysiologic and psychological reasons. Despite this experience, he continued to smoke about 30 cigarettes a day, a habit he started when he joined the Navy at the age of 19.

Since the episode 4 years ago, however, the patient's medical history had been essentially unremarkable. As instructed, he scheduled an appointment with his doctor on a regular basis, twice a year. Most of the time he demonstrated a productive cough and wheezing. The patient was generally on several medications, including daily dosages of antibiotics, xanthines, expectorants, and aerosolized sympathomimetics. Three or four times a week, for about 30 minutes, the patient also performed a number of the breathing exercises previously shown to him by the pulmonary rehabilitation team.

He had worked as a janitor for over 30 years in the local public school system. At the time of this admission he was 7 months away from his retirement party. Even though he had had chronic bronchitis and emphysema for many years, he had always been considered a reliable, hardworking employee by the school administration and fellow workers. Although he often went to work feeling less than well, he could always finish out the day with no major problems. He seldom complained about his health in an effort not to draw attention to himself.

About 4 days before the present admission, however, he started to find it difficult to make it through the entire work day. He told his wife that he thought he was getting the flu, with symptoms of fatigue, chills, and a cough that was getting worse and more productive. He nevertheless continued to go to work each day and made it to the end of the week. At home on Saturday, 2 hours before admission, he suddenly became very short of breath with minimal exertion. At one point he was unable to climb the stairs to his bedroom without stopping several times to rest. Concerned, his wife helped him into the car and drove him to the hospital.

PHYSICAL EXAMINATION

The patient was in obvious respiratory distress. He was sitting in a wheelchair, with his arms anchored to the arms of the chair, using his accessory muscles of respiration.

He was a thin but well-nourished man. His skin appeared cyanotic, and his fingers were clubbed. He was pursed-lip breathing, and his chest was barrel shaped. He demonstrated a frequent, strong cough productive of large amounts of thick, yellow and green sputum. He stated that he had been coughing so much and so hard that his chest hurt around his left collar bone area.

His vital signs were blood pressure 145/85, heart rate 94 bpm, respiratory rate 20/min, and temperature 37.9° C (100.3° F). Palpation of the chest was unremarkable. Percussion revealed hyperresonant notes bilaterally. Auscultation revealed diminished breath sounds and rhonchi throughout both lung fields. His heart sounds were diminished. Expiration took three times as long as inspiration.

His last pulmonary function study (PFT), taken about 6 months before at his last doctor's appointment, showed that he had a moderate-to-severe obstructive disorder. His chest x-ray film in the emergency room revealed dark, translucent lung fields, depressed and flattened hemidiaphragms, and a long, narrow heart. A small anterior pneumothorax (about 10%) was also noted between the second and third ribs. His arterial blood gas values on room air were pH 7.53, $Paco_2$ 48 mm Hg, HCO_3^- 38 mmol/L, and Pao_2 57 mm Hg. His baseline arterial blood gas values at his last medical appointment were pH 7.42, $Paco_2$ 69 mm Hg, HCO_3^- 41 mmol/L, Pao_2 74 mm Hg. The physician ordered guaifenesin (Robitussin), theophylline (Theo-Dur), bed rest with limited physical activity, and a respiratory care consult.

RESPONSE 1

On the basis of the above information, write your SOAP in the following space.

S _____

O _____

A _____

● P _____
_____
_____
_____
_____
_____

3 HOURS LATER

The patient's primary nurse called a physician and paged respiratory care stat. A repeat chest x-ray film made by portable machine was also requested. The patient's respiratory distress had obviously worsened. The nurse stated that the patient had just pressed his bedside buzzer requesting help for his breathing. As the respiratory therapist walked into the patient's room, the patient stated that he felt "like hell."

He appeared cyanotic and was pursed-lip breathing and perspiring. He demonstrated a frequent but weak cough, and when he did cough, he would pull his left arm to his side in an effort to brace himself. Although he expectorated only a small amount of sputum, he sounded "full." Rhonchi could be heard without the aid of a stethoscope. The sputum he did produce was still thick and yellow-green. His left anterior chest appeared hyperinflated and fixed compared to the right.

His vital signs were blood pressure 95/55, heart rate 125 bpm, and weak, and respiratory rate 28/min and shallow. Palpation of the chest was unremarkable. Percussion revealed hyperresonant notes bilaterally. Auscultation revealed diminished breath sounds and rhonchi throughout in the right lung and no breath sounds whatsoever over the left lung fields. Diminished heart sounds could be heard to the right of the sternum. His arterial blood gas values were pH 7.24, $Paco_2$ 103 mm Hg, HCO_3^- 43 mmol/L, and Pao_2 37 mm Hg. His hemoglobin oxygen saturation measured by pulse oximetry (Spo_2) was 62%.

The chest x-ray film showed that the patient's original small, left-sided pneumothorax had dramatically increased: The entire left lung was now collapsed; the left hemidiaphragm was significantly lower than the right; the mediastinum had shifted to the right; and patches of atelectasis could be seen throughout the right lung.

The attending physician, along with a physician's assistant, inserted a chest tube in the left pleural cavity and began suction with negative pressure of −10 cm H_2O. The physician stated that in light of the problems the patient had in the past, he did not want to commit the patient to a ventilator. He requested a respiratory care consult, with a chest x-ray film taken by portable machine to follow the first respiratory therapy treatments by 30 minutes.

RESPONSE 2

On the basis of the above information, write your SOAP in the following space.

S _____
_____

O _____
● _____
_____

_____

_____

_____

_____

A _____

_____

_____

_____

_____

_____

_____

P _____

_____

_____

_____

_____

30 MINUTES LATER

Although the patient was still in respiratory distress, he had improved. The chest x-ray film showed that his left lung had reexpanded about 75%. The right lung was translucent with no signs of atelectasis. The mediastinum had moved back to its normal position. The patient stated that he was feeling better. He still appeared cyanotic, and he was pursed-lip breathing. He was still using his accessory muscles of respiration. Although he was still perspiring, it was less than 30 minutes earlier.

No spontaneous cough or sputum production was observed at this time. However, auscultation revealed diminished breath sounds and rhonchi over the right lung field. Breath sounds were diminished over the left lung area. His vital signs were blood pressure 145/85, heart rate 105 bpm, and respiratory rate 22/min. He was no longer cyanotic. Palpation of the chest was unremarkable. Percussion revealed hyperresonant notes bilaterally. Diminished heart sounds were no longer heard over the right lung area. His arterial blood gas values were pH 7.35, $Paco_2$ 85 mm Hg, HCO_3^- 41 mmol/L, and Pao_2 64 mm Hg. His Spo_2 was 90%.

RESPONSE 3

On the basis of the above information, write your SOAP in the following space.

S _____

_____

O _____

_____

A

P

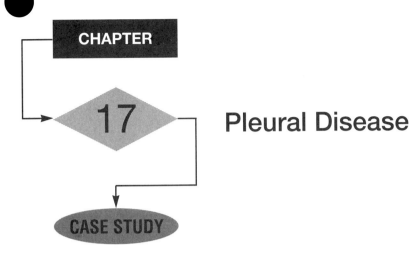

CHAPTER

17 Pleural Disease

CASE STUDY

ADMITTING HISTORY

Against her doctor's advice, this 38-year-old white woman discharged herself from the hospital about 2 months before the present admission. At that time she had been admitted for right lower lobe pneumonia, which was described as severe. After 5 days of treatment she became angry because she was not allowed to smoke. She was a long-time, three-pack-per-day smoker. When a nurse found her smoking in her hospital bed with a 2 L/min oxygen nasal cannula, her cigarettes and matches were quickly confiscated.

The patient became upset. She told her doctor that this was the last straw and that she was going to walk out of the hospital on her own. Her doctor wanted her to remain so that she could do a thorough follow-up for what she described as a "spot" on her lower right lung. The patient promised that she would make an appointment at the doctor's office in a week or so. She then got dressed and left. Two days after she left the hospital, however, she felt so much better that she decided the spot on her lung was not an issue to be concerned about. The patient told her friends that smoking one pack of cigarettes made her feel better than 5 days' worth of nurses, doctors, and hospitals.

On the day of the present admission the patient appeared at the doctor's office without an appointment. She told the receptionist that something was very wrong. She thought that she had the flu and that it had been getting progressively worse over the last 4 days. At this time, she could only speak in short sentences and was unable to inhale deeply. Seeing that the patient was in obvious respiratory distress, the nurse interrupted the doctor. Within 5 minutes the doctor had the patient transported and admitted to the hospital a few blocks away.

ADMITTING HISTORY

The patient appeared malnourished, had poor personal hygiene, and had yellow tobacco stains around her fingers. She appeared in moderate-to-severe respiratory distress. Her skin was cyanotic, and her shirt was wet from perspiration. She demonstrated an occasional hacking, nonproductive cough. She stated that she could not take a deep breath and that maybe it was from that spot on her lung.

Her vital signs were blood pressure 146/92, heart rate 112 bpm, and respiratory rate 36/min and shallow. She was slightly febrile with an oral temperature of 37.7°C

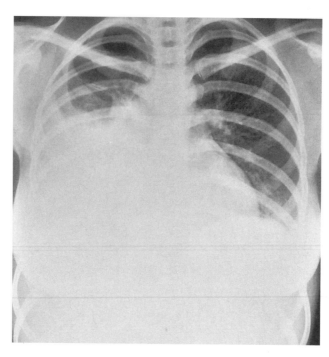

Fig. 17-1

(99.8° F). Palpation showed the trachea was slightly shifted to the left. Dull percussion notes were found over the right middle and right lower lobes. Auscultation revealed normal vesicular breath sounds over the left lung fields and upper right lobe. No breath sounds could be heard over the right middle and right lower lobes.

The patient's chest x-ray film showed a large, right-sided pleural effusion. There was blunting of the right costophrenic angle; the right hemidiaphragm was depressed; and the right middle and lower lung lobes were partially collapsed and showed greater density consistent with pneumonia. The patient's trachea and mediastinum were slightly shifted to the left (Fig. 17-1). The patient's arterial blood gas values on a 3 L/min O_2 cannula were pH 7.53, $Paco_2$ 24 mm Hg, HCO_3^- 19 mmol/L, and Pao_2 37 mm Hg. The patient's oxygen saturation measured by pulse oximetry (Spo_2) was 74%. The doctor, assisted by the respiratory therapist, performed a thoracentesis on the patient at the bedside. A little over 2 L of yellow fluid was withdrawn. The patient was then started on intravenous antibiotics. A chest x-ray film taken by a portable machine was ordered, and a respiratory care consult was requested.

RESPONSE 1

On the basis of the above information, write your SOAP in the following space.

S _____

_____

O _____

_____

_____

_____

_____

_____

_____

_____

A _____

_____

_____

_____

_____

_____

_____

_____

P _____

_____

_____

_____

_____

_____

_____

3 HOURS AFTER ADMISSION

At this time the patient was sitting up in bed and stated that although she was feeling better, she did not feel great. She still had an occasional dry sounding, nonproductive cough. Her skin was pale and cyanotic. She was no longer perspiring as she was when she was first admitted. Her vital signs were blood pressure 135/85, heart rate 100 bpm, and respiratory rate 24/min. Her respiratory efforts, however, no longer appeared to be shallow. Her temperature was normal at this time. Palpation was not remarkable. Dull percussion notes were found over the right middle and right lower lobes. Normal vesicular breath sounds were heard over the left lung and over the upper right lung. Loud bronchial breath sounds could be heard over the right middle and right lower lobes.

The patient's chest x-ray film showed a small, right-sided pleural effusion. There was still increased opacity in the right middle and lower lung consistent with pneumonia. The patient's trachea and mediastinum were now in their normal positions. The patient's arterial blood gas values were pH 7.52, $Paco_2$ 29 mm Hg, HCO_3^- 22 mmol/L, and Pao_2 57 mm Hg. The patient's Spo_2 was 89%.

RESPONSE 2

On the basis of the above information, write your SOAP in the following space.

S _____

_____

_____

O _____

_____

_____

_____

_____

_____

_____

A _____

_____

_____

_____

_____

_____

P _____

_____

_____

_____

_____

5 HOURS AFTER ADMISSION

Thirty minutes before the respiratory care practitioner planned to call the physician to present an update of the patient's respiratory status, the practitioner prepared a full SOAP. The patient was in semi-Fowler's position. She appeared relaxed and alert. She stated that she had finally caught her breath. Although she still appeared pale, she did not look cyanotic. No spontaneous cough was observed at this time.

Her vital signs were blood pressure 128/79, heart rate 88 bpm, respiratory rate 16/min, and temperature normal. Palpation of the chest was not remarkable. Dull percussion notes were found over the right middle and right lower lobes. Normal vesicular breath sounds were heard over the left lung and over the right upper lobe. Bronchial breath sounds could be heard over the right middle and right lower lobes. No current chest x-ray film was available. The patient's arterial blood gas values were pH 7.45, $Paco_2$ 36 mm Hg, HCO_3^- 24 mmol/L, and Pao_2 77 mm Hg. The patient's Spo_2 was 92%.

RESPONSE 3

On the basis of the above information, write your SOAP in the following space.

S _____
_____
_____

O _____
_____
_____
_____
_____
_____
_____
_____

A _____
_____
_____
_____
_____
_____
_____

P _____
_____
_____
_____
_____

18 Kyphoscoliosis

ADMITTING HISTORY

Idiopathic kyphoscoliosis began to develop in this 62-year-old white woman when she was 6 years old. She lived in the mountains of Virginia all her life, with her parents and later her two older sisters. Although she wore several different body braces up until she was 17 years old, her disorder was classified as severe by the time she was 15 years old. The doctors, who were few and far between, always told her that she would have to learn to live with her condition the best she could, and as a general rule she did.

She finished high school with no other remarkable physical or personal problems. She was well liked by her classmates. She was actively involved in the school newspaper and art club. After graduation she continued to live with her parents for a few more years. At the age of 21 she moved in with her two older sisters, who were buying a large farm house near a small but popular tourist town. All three sisters made various arts and crafts, which they sold at local tourist shops. The patient's physical disability and general health were relatively stable until she was about 40 years old. Around that time the patient started to experience frequent episodes of dyspnea, coughing, and sputum production. As the years progressed, her baseline condition was marked by more and more severe dyspnea.

Because the sisters rarely ventured to the city, the patient's medical resources were described as poor until she was introduced to a new social worker at a nearby church. The church had just become part of an outreach program based in a large city nearby. The social worker was charmed by the patient and fascinated by the beauty of the colorful quilts she made.

The social worker, however, was also concerned by the patient's limited ability to move because of her severe chest deformity. In addition, the social worker felt the patient's cough sounded very bad. She noted that the patient appeared grayish blue, weak, and ill. The sisters told the social worker that their sister had had a bad cold for about 6 months. It took much urging, but the social worker was able to convince the patient to travel, accompanied by her sisters, to the city to see a doctor at a large hospital associated with the church outreach program. Upon arrival the patient was admitted to the hospital. The sisters stayed in a nearby hotel room, which was provided by the hospital.

PHYSICAL EXAMINATION

The patient appeared to be a well-nourished white woman with severe kyphoscoliosis. The lateral curvature of the spine was twisted significantly to the patient's left. She looked older than her stated age, and she was in obvious respiratory distress. The patient stated that she was having trouble breathing. Her skin was cyanotic. She had digital clubbing, and her neck veins were distended, especially on the right side. The patient demonstrated a frequent but adequate cough. During each coughing episode the patient expectorated a moderate amount of thick, yellow sputum.

It was also noted that when the patient generated a strong cough, a large unilateral "bulge" appeared at the right anterolateral base of the patient's neck, just posterior to the clavicle. The patient referred to the bulge as her "Dizzy Gillespie" pouch. The doctor felt that the bulge was a result of the severe kyphoscoliosis, which had in turn stretched and weakened the suprapleural membrane that normally restricts and contains the parietal pleura at the apex of the lung. Because of the weakening of the suprapleural membrane, any time the patient produced a Valsalva maneuver for any reason (e.g., for coughing), the increased intrapleural pressure herniated the suprapleural membrane outward. Despite its odd appearance, the doctor did not feel the bulge was a serious concern at this time.

The patient's vital signs were blood pressure 160/100, heart rate 90 bpm, respiratory rate 18/min, and oral temperature 36.3° C (97.4° F). Palpation revealed a trachea deviated to the right. Dull percussion notes were produced over both lungs. Crackles and rhonchi were heard over both lungs. A pulmonary function study (PFT) conducted that morning showed vital capacity (VC), functional residual capacity (FRC), and residual volume (RV) to be between 45% and 50% of predicted.

Although the patient's electrolytes were all normal, her hematocrit was 58%, and her hemoglobin was 18 g/dl. A chest x-ray film revealed a severe thoracic and spinous deformity, a mediastinal shift, an enlarged heart with prominent pulmonary artery segments bilaterally, and bilateral infiltrates in the lung bases consistent with pneumonia and atelectasis (Fig. 18-1). The patient's arterial blood gas values on room air were pH 7.52, $Paco_2$ 58 mm Hg, HCO_3^- 42 mmol/L, and Pao_2 49 mm Hg. Her oxygen saturation measured by pulse oximetry (Spo_2) was 78%. The physician requested a respiratory care consult and stated that mechanical ventilation was not an option at this time per the patient's request and his knowledge of the case.

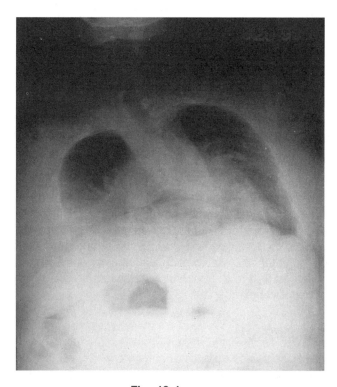

Fig. 18-1

RESPONSE 1

On the basis of the above information, write your SOAP in the following space.

S _____

_____

O _____

_____

_____

_____

_____

_____

_____

_____

A _____

_____

_____

_____

_____

_____

_____

_____

P _____

_____

_____

_____

_____

_____

_____

_____

10 HOURS FOLLOWING ADMISSION

The physician had trouble titrating the patient's cardiac drugs and decided to insert a pulmonary artery catheter, central venous catheter, and an arterial line. Because of the patient's cardiac problems, several medical students, respiratory therapists, nurses, and doctors were constantly in and out of the patient's room performing and assisting in various procedures. As a result it was difficult to work with the patient for any length of time, and the intensity of respiratory care was less than desirable.

Eventually the patient's cardiac status stabilized, and the physician requested an update on the patient's pulmonary condition.

The respiratory therapist working on the pulmonary consult team found the patient in extreme respiratory distress. The patient was sitting up in bed, appeared frightened, and stated that she was extremely short of breath. Both of the patient's sisters were in the room; one sister was putting cold towels on the patient's face, and the other sister was holding the patient's hands. Both of the sisters were crying softly.

The patient's skin was cyanotic, and perspiration could be seen on her face. Her neck veins were still distended. She demonstrated a weak, spontaneous cough. Although no sputum was noted, she sounded congested when she coughed. Dull percussion notes, crackles, and rhonchi were still present throughout both lungs. Her vital signs were blood pressure 180/120, heart rate 130 bpm, respiratory rate 26/min, and rectal temperature 37.8° C (100° F).

Several of the patient's hemodynamic indices were elevated: CVP, RAP, $\overline{PA}$, RVSWI, and PVR.* All other hemodynamic indices were normal. Her oxygenation indices were increased $\dot{Q}s/\dot{Q}t$ and O_2ER and decreased D_{O_2} and $S\bar{v}_{O_2}$. Her $\dot{V}_{O_2}$ and $C(a-\bar{v})_{O_2}$ were normal.† No recent chest x-ray film was available. Her arterial blood gas values were pH 7.57, Pa_{CO_2} 49 mm Hg, HCO_3^- 40 mmol/L, and Pa_{O_2} 43 mm Hg. Her Sp_{O_2} was 76%.

---

*CVP = central venous pressure, RAP = right atrial pressure, $\overline{PA}$ = mean pulmonary artery pressure, RVSWI = right ventricular stroke work index, PVR = pulmonary vascular resistance.

†$\dot{Q}s/\dot{Q}T$ = cardiac output shunted per total cardiac output, O_2ER = oxygen extraction ratio, D_{O_2} = total oxygen delivery, $S\bar{v}_{O_2}$ = mixed venous oxygen saturation, $\dot{V}_{O_2}$ = oxygen consumption per unit time, $C(a-\bar{v})_{O_2}$ = arterial − mixed venous difference in oxygen concentration.

RESPONSE 2

On the basis of the above information, write your SOAP in the following space.

S _____

_____

O _____

_____

_____

_____

_____

_____

_____

A _____

_____

_____

_____

●

P _____

_____

_____

_____

_____

_____

_____

24 HOURS AFTER ADMISSION

At this time the respiratory care practitioner found the patient watching the morning news on television with her two sisters. The patient was in semi-Fowler's position and was eating the last few bites of her breakfast. The patient stated that she felt "so much better" and that "finally I have enough wind to eat some food."

Although the patient's skin still appeared pale and cyanotic, she did not look so bad as she had the day before. On request, she produced a strong cough. She expectorated a small amount of white sputum. Her vital signs were blood pressure 140/85, heart rate 83 bpm, respiratory rate 14/min, and temperature normal. Chest assessment findings showed crackles, rhonchi, and dull percussion notes over both lung fields. The rhonchi were less intense, however, than the day before.

Although the patient's hemodynamic and oxygenation indices were better than the day before, there was still room for improvement. Her hemodynamic parameters still revealed an elevated CVP, RAP, $\overline{PA}$, RVSWI, and PVR. All other hemodynamic indices were normal. Her oxygenation indices still showed an increased $\dot{Q}s/\dot{Q}t$ and O_2ER and a decreased D_{O_2} and $S\bar{v}_{O_2}$. Her $\dot{V}_{O_2}$ and $C(a-\bar{v})_{O_2}$ were normal. The patient's chest x-ray film taken earlier that morning showed some clearing of the pneumonia and atelectasis described when the patient was first admitted. Her arterial blood gas values were pH 7.45, Pa_{CO_2} 73 mm Hg, HCO_3^- 48 mmol/L, and Pa_{O_2} 68 mm Hg. Her Sp_{O_2} was 93%.

RESPONSE 3

On the basis of the above information, write your SOAP in the following space.

S _____

O _____

_____

_____

_____

_____

_____

A _____

_____

_____

_____

_____

_____

_____

_____

P _____

_____

_____

_____

_____

_____

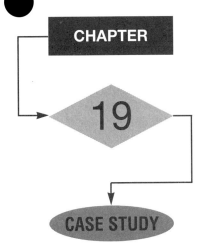

PART VII
ENVIRONMENTAL LUNG DISEASES

CHAPTER

19   Pneumoconiosis

CASE STUDY

ADMITTING HISTORY

This 72-year-old black man was well known to the treating hospital, having received care there for over 12 years. While in the U.S. Navy during the Second World War, he worked on the East Coast in the ship construction industry. After his discharge in 1945 he returned to his home in Mississippi for about 6 months; he then moved to Detroit, Michigan, and began to work for an automobile manufacturer. His primary job for the next 20 years was undercoating automobiles.

In the early 1970s the patient was transferred to a nearby automotive plant, where he worked on an assembly line, fastening bumpers and chrome trim to cars. He was well liked by his fellow workers and was considered a hard worker by the administration. When he retired in 1980, he was one of four supervisors in charge of the chrome trim assembly line.

Although the patient had been a two-pack-a-day smoker for more than 40 years, his health was essentially unremarkable until about 4 years before he retired. At that time he started to experience periods of coughing, dyspnea, and weakness. A complete examination provided by the company concluded that the patient had moderate pneumoconiosis.

On the basis of the patient's work history, the doctor speculated that the pneumoconiosis was caused by asbestos fibers. This was later confirmed with a Perl stain of sputum, and the diagnosis of asbestosis was put in the patient's chart. Just before the patient retired, his pulmonary function studies showed a mild-to-moderate combined restrictive and obstructive disorder.

Although the patient was able to enjoy a couple of relatively good years of retirement with his wife, after that his health rapidly declined. His cough and dyspnea quickly became a daily problem. Despite his deteriorating health, the patient continued to smoke. When he was 68 years old, he was hospitalized for 8 days for pneumonia and severe respiratory distress. When he was discharged at that time, his pulmonary function studies still showed a moderate-to-severe restrictive and obstructive disorder. He started using oxygen at home on a regular basis.

Ten months before the current admission the patient was hospitalized for congestive heart failure. He was treated aggressively and sent home within 5 days. At discharge his pulmonary function study results showed that he had a severe restrictive and obstructive respiratory disorder. His arterial blood gases on 1 L/min oxygen by nasal cannula were pH 7.38, $Paco_2$ 86 mm Hg, HCO_3^- 46 mmol/L, and Pao_2 63 mm Hg.

Three hours before this admission the patient woke up from an afternoon nap extremely short of breath. His wife stated that he coughed almost continuously and that he had difficulty speaking. She took his temperature and found it to be 38° C (100.4° F). Concerned, the patient's wife drove him to the hospital emergency room.

PHYSICAL EXAMINATION

As the patient was wheeled into the emergency room, he appeared nervous, weak, and in obvious respiratory distress. His breathing pattern was classified as tachypnea by the emergency room doctor. He was on a 1.5 L/min oxygen cannula, which was connected to an E-tank that was attached to the wheelchair. His skin felt damp and clammy. He appeared pale and cyanotic. His neck veins were distended, and his fingers and toes were clubbed. He had a frequent but weak cough productive of a moderate amount of thick, whitish yellow secretions. He had 3+ peripheral edema of the ankles and feet. He said this was the worst his breathing had ever been.

The patient's vital signs were blood pressure 182/106, heart rate 108 bpm, respiratory rate 32/min, and oral temperature 38.3° C (100.8° F). Palpation of the chest was negative. Percussion produced bilateral dull notes in the lung bases. Wheezing, rhonchi, and crackles were auscultated throughout both lungs. A pleural friction rub could be heard over the right middle lobe between the sixth and seventh ribs and between the anterior axillary line and midaxillary line.

The patient's lower lobes had a diffuse ground-glass appearance on the chest x-ray film. Also seen were irregularly shaped opacities in the right and left lower pleural spaces that were identified by the radiologist as calcified pleural plaques. A possible infiltrate consistent with pneumonia also was seen in the right middle lobe. The chest x-ray film also disclosed that the right side of the heart was moderately enlarged (Fig. 19-1). His arterial blood gas values on a 1.5 L/min O_2 cannula were pH 7.56, $Paco_2$ 51 mm Hg, HCO_3^- 38 mmol/L, and Pao_2 47 mm Hg.

The physician started the patient on intravenous (IV) furosemide (Lasix) to treat the patient's cor pulmonale and began an antibiotic for the patient's pneumonia. Respiratory care was called to obtain a sputum culture, to perform a respiratory care evaluation, and to outline further respiratory therapy. The physician said she did not want to commit the patient to a ventilator unless it was absolutely necessary.

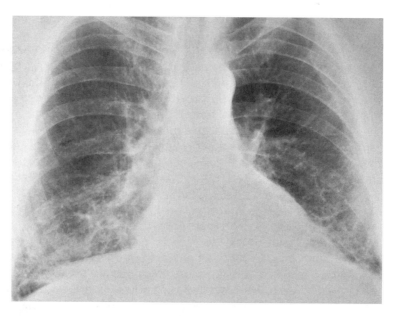

Fig. 19-1

RESPONSE 1

On the basis of the above information, write your SOAP in the following space.

S _____

_____

O _____

_____

_____

_____

_____

_____

A _____

_____

_____

_____

_____

_____

_____

P _____

_____

_____

_____

_____

_____

THE NEXT MORNING

Throughout the night the patient's condition remained unstable. He continued to cough frequently but was not able to expectorate secretions very well on his own. When the therapist assisted the patient in his cough effort, a moderate amount of thick, white and yellow sputum was produced. Even though he was conscious, alert, and able to follow simple directions, he did not answer any questions asked by the respiratory practitioner regarding his breathing.

His skin was cold and damp to the touch, and he appeared short of breath. His color was improved, but he was still pale and cyanotic. His neck veins were still distended, although not so severely as when he was first admitted, and edema of his ankles and feet could still be seen. The patient's vital signs were blood pressure 192/108, heart rate 113 bpm, respiratory rate 34/min, and temperature 38° C (100.4° F). Palpation of the chest was negative.

Dull percussion notes were elicited over the lung bases. Wheezing, rhonchi, and crackles continued to be auscultated throughout both lungs. A pleural friction rub could still be heard over the right middle lung lobe between the sixth and seventh ribs and between the anterior axillary line and midaxillary line. No recent chest x-ray film was available. His arterial blood gas values were pH 7.57, $Paco_2$ 47 mm Hg, HCO_3^- 36 mmol/L, and Pao_2 40 mm Hg. His oxygen saturation measured by pulse oximetry (Spo_2) was 77%.

RESPONSE 2

On the basis of the above information, write your SOAP in the following space.

S _____

_____

O _____

_____

_____

_____

_____

_____

A _____

_____

_____

_____

_____

_____

_____

_____

P _____

_____

_____

_____

_____

_____

20 HOURS LATER

At 0615 the alarm on the patient's ECG monitor sounded. The ECG strip showed several premature ventricular contractions followed by ventricular flutter and fibrillation. The head nurse called for a code blue. Cardiopulmonary resuscitation was started immediately. Epinephrine and dobutamine were administered through the patient's IV line. Twelve minutes into the code the patient had a normal sinus rhythm. Spontaneous respirations were absent.

The patient was intubated, transferred to the intensive care unit (ICU), and placed on a mechanical ventilator. The patient's initial ventilator settings were control mode, 12 breaths per minute, F_{IO_2} 1.0, pressure support +4 cm H_2O, and +10 cm H_2O positive end expiratory pressure (PEEP). The patient's cardiopulmonary status continued to be unstable. Premature ventricular contractions were frequently seen on the ECG monitor. A pulmonary artery catheter and arterial line were inserted.

The patient's skin was pale, cyanotic, and clammy. His neck veins were still distended, and his ankles and feet were swollen. The patient's vital signs were blood pressure 135/90, heart rate 84 bpm, and temperature 38.3° C (100.8° F). Palpation of the chest wall was negative. Dull percussion notes were produced over the lung bases. Wheezing, rhonchi, and crackles continued to be auscultated throughout both lungs. Thick, greenish yellow sputum was frequently suctioned from the patient's endotracheal tube.

A pleural friction rub could still be heard over the right middle lung lobe between the sixth and seventh ribs and between the anterior axillary line and midaxillary line. A chest x-ray film had been taken but had not yet been interpreted by the radiologist. The patient's hemodynamic indices were elevated CVP, RAP, $\overline{PA}$, RVSWI, and PVR.* All other hemodynamic values were normal. His arterial blood gas values were pH 7.53, Pa_{CO_2} 56 mm Hg, HCO_3^- 38 mmol/L, Pa_{O_2} 246 mm Hg. His Sp_{O_2} was 98%.

*CVP = central venous pressure, RAP = right atrial pressure, $\overline{PA}$ = mean pulmonary artery pressure, RVSWI = right ventricular stroke work index, PVR = pulmonary vascular resistance.

RESPONSE 3

On the basis of the above data, write your SOAP in the following space.

S ___

O ___

A ___

P

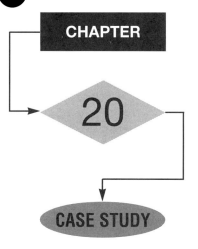

PART VIII
NEOPLASTIC DISEASES

CHAPTER

20 Cancer of the Lungs

CASE STUDY

ADMITTING HISTORY

This 66-year-old retired white man lived with his wife in a small, two-bedroom ranch house in Peoria, Illinois, during the summer months. During the rest of the year, they lived in a 22-foot trailer in a retirement park just outside of Las Vegas, Nevada. The trailer park was conveniently located on the casinos' shuttle bus route; a bus came by at the top of every hour.

Both the patient and his wife were described by their children as addicted gamblers. They gambled almost every day of the year. During the summer months they played keno and blackjack on the Par-A-Dice Riverboat Casino, which was docked along the shores of the Illinois river in downtown East Peoria. While in Las Vegas, they played bingo, blackjack, and the slot machines at several different casinos. They would dress in matching warm-up suits, ride the bus to one of the casinos, and gamble until 10 or 11 PM every day.

Their children, who were adults with their own families, homes, and jobs in the Peoria area, were concerned about their parents' gambling. They had tried to no avail to get their parents to see a compulsive-gambling therapist, who was actually provided by the Par-A-Dice Riverboat Casino.

Their children's concern was justified. Their parents were always gambling on a shoestring budget. Although they still owned their trailer and small home in Peoria, within the last 2 years they had gambled away most of their life savings, which included stocks, bonds, and mutual funds. Because they had let their health insurance premium lapse, their policy had recently been canceled. They still received a small monthly pension check, however, and some social security.

Before he retired the patient worked for 17 years as a boiler tender for Methodist Hospital in Peoria. He was also a part-time fireman. For over 52 years he had smoked between two and a half and three packs of unfiltered cigarettes a day. While in Las Vegas about 3 months earlier the patient became aware that he was having periods of dyspnea, coughing, and weakness. His cough was productive of small amounts of clear secretions. It was also around this time that his wife first noticed that his voice sounded hoarse.

Even though he missed several days of gambling and remained in bed because of weakness, he did not seek medical attention. He hated doctors and felt he only had a bad cold and the flu anyway. When he returned to Peoria for the summer, however, the children became concerned and insisted that he see a doctor. Despite

121

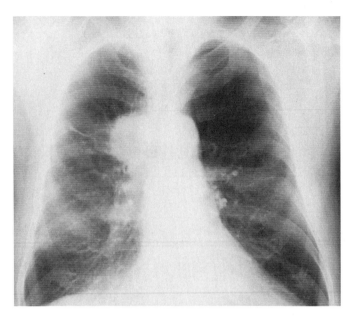

Fig. 20-1

the patient's lack of health insurance, a full diagnostic workup was ordered by two medical students from the University of Illinois, who were working as a team.

A pulmonary function study (PFT) showed that the patient had a restrictive and obstructive pulmonary disorder. Computed tomography scanning (CT scan) showed that the patient had several masses, ranging from 2 to 5 cm in diameter, in the right and left mediastinum in the hilar regions. The masses, especially on the right side, could also be seen clearly on the patient's posteroanterior chest radiograph (Fig. 20-1). Both the CT scan and the chest x-ray film showed an increased opacity consistent with atelectasis of the left lower lobe as well.

A fiberoptic bronchoscopic examination was conducted by the pulmonary physician with the assistance of a respiratory therapist trained in special procedures. It showed several large, protruding bronchial masses in the second- and third-generation bronchi of the right lung and the second-, third-, and fourth-generation bronchi of the left lung. During the bronchoscopy, several mucus plugs were suctioned out. Biopsy of three of the larger tumors was positive for squamous cell bronchogenic carcinoma, and the patient was admitted to the hospital.

The physician told the patient that he had cancer and that his prognosis was poor. Treatment, at best, would be palliative. The patient asked what the odds were on his life expectancy. The physician stated that there was only about a 50% chance that he would live longer than 6 to 8 weeks. Surgery was out of the question. In the interim, however, the physician promised to do what was possible to make the patient comfortable. The physician outlined a treatment plan of radiation therapy and chemotherapy and requested a respiratory care consult.

PHYSICAL EXAMINATION

The respiratory care practitioner reviewed the above information in the patient's chart. The patient was found sitting up in bed in obvious respiratory distress. He appeared weak. His skin was cyanotic, and his face, arms, and chest were damp with perspiration. Wheezing could be heard with the aid of a stethoscope. He stated in a hoarse voice that he had coughed up a cup of sputum since breakfast 2 hours ago. He demonstrated a weak cough every few minutes or so. His cough was productive of copious blood-streaked sputum. The viscosity of the sputum was "thin." After each coughing episode he stated that he wanted a cigarette and then laughed.

His vital signs were blood pressure 155/85, heart rate 90 bpm, respiratory rate 22/min, and temperature normal. Palpation was not remarkable. Percussion produced dull notes over the left lower lobe. On auscultation, rhonchi, wheezing, and crackles could be heard throughout both lung fields. His arterial blood gas values on a 2 L/min oxygen nasal cannula were pH 7.51, $Paco_2$ 29 mm Hg, HCO_3^- 22 mmol/L, and Pao_2 66 mm Hg. His oxygen saturation measured by pulse oximetry (Spo_2) was 92%.

RESPONSE 1

On the basis of the above information, write your SOAP in the following space.

S _____

_____

O _____

_____

_____

_____

_____

_____

_____

A _____

_____

_____

_____

_____

_____

_____

_____

P _____

_____

_____

_____

_____

_____

_____

3 DAYS AFTER ADMISSION

During morning rounds the patient was evaluated by respiratory care. After reviewing the patient's chart, the practitioner went to the patient's bedside. The patient was not tolerating the chemotherapy well. He had been vomiting off and on for the past

10 hours and was still in obvious respiratory distress. He appeared cyanotic and tired, and his hospital gown was wet from perspiration. His cough was still weak and productive of large amounts of moderately thick clear and white sputum. He stated in a hoarse voice that he still was not breathing very well.

His vital signs were blood pressure 166/90, heart rate 95 bpm, respiratory rate 28/min, and temperature normal. Dull percussion notes were elicited over both the right and left lower lobes. Rhonchi, wheezing, and crackles were auscultated throughout both lung fields. His arterial blood gas values were pH 7.55, Pa_{CO_2} 25 mm Hg, HCO_3^- 20 mmol/L, and Pa_{O_2} 53 mm Hg. His Sp_{O_2} was 88%.

RESPONSE 2

On the basis of the above information, write your SOAP in the following space.

S _____

_____

_____

O _____

_____

_____

_____

_____

_____

_____

A _____

_____

_____

_____

_____

_____

_____

_____

P _____

_____

_____

_____

_____

_____

_____

16 DAYS AFTER ADMISSION

Although it had been the physician's original intention and hope to discharge the patient soon, it was difficult to get the patient stabilized for any length of time. Over the past 2 weeks the patient had continued to be nauseated on a daily basis. He did, however, have occasional periods of relief in his ability to breathe, but he generally was in respiratory distress.

On this day the respiratory therapist observed and collected the following clinical data: The patient was lying in bed in the supine position. His eyes were closed, and he was unresponsive to the therapist's questions. The patient was in obvious respiratory distress. He appeared pale, cyanotic, and diaphoretic. No cough was observed at this time, but rhonchi could easily be heard from across the patient's room. The nurse in the patient's room stated that the doctor had earlier called the rhonchi a "death rattle."

The patient's vital signs were blood pressure 170/105, heart rate 110 bpm, respiratory rate 11/min and shallow, and temperature normal. Percussion was not performed. Rhonchi, wheezing, and crackles were heard throughout both lung fields. His arterial blood gas values were pH 7.28, $Paco_2$ 63 mm Hg, HCO_3^- 27 mmol/L, and Pao_2 66 mm Hg. His Spo_2 was 90%.

RESPONSE 3

On the basis of the above information, write your SOAP in the following space.

S _____

_____

O _____

_____

_____

_____

_____

_____

_____

A _____

_____

_____

_____

_____

_____

_____

_____

P _____

_____

_____

_____

_____

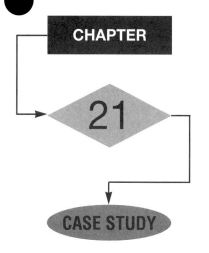

CHAPTER

21

CASE STUDY

Adult Respiratory Distress Syndrome

ADMITTING HISTORY

This 32-year-old man was involved in an automobile accident on the way to work during an ice storm. His car hit a patch of ice, spun out of control, and hit a cement bridge support. It took a 911 team 90 minutes to extricate him from the car. He was stabilized at the accident site and then transported to the hospital. Although he was unconscious, he started to move and speak en route to the hospital. His speech was incoherent.

On admission he was hypotensive, conscious, and complaining of severe pain. When he was asked to identify specific pain sites, he stated that his whole body hurt. He had numerous facial lacerations and several broken teeth. A zygomatic arch was broken, and his right maxilla was fractured. He had a compound fracture of the left humerus, a Colles fracture of the left radius, and several simple fractures of the first, second, and third phalanges on his left hand. A large bruise in the shape of a car steering wheel could easily be observed over his anterior chest. He had a splintered fracture of his right tibia and fibula. Although the chest x-ray film made in the emergency room showed no rib fractures, bilateral patchy infiltrates could be seen throughout both lungs.

He was taken to surgery, where maxillofacial, plastic, and orthopedic surgeons worked to treat his multiple injuries. The patient was in the operating room for 16 hours. His surgery was described as successful, and the long-term prognosis was believed to be good. He was in the postoperative recovery room for 2 hours with no remarkable problems and was then transferred to the surgical intensive care unit (ICU).

On arrival in the ICU the patient was breathing on his own, receiving supplemental oxygen via a 2 L/min nasal cannula. His general cardiopulmonary status was stable, and his recovery for the first 24 hours was as expected. At that time, however, the patient started to show signs of respiratory distress, and the attending physician ordered a respiratory care consultation.

PHYSICAL EXAMINATION

The respiratory therapist assigned to evaluate and treat the patient gathered the following clinical information: On inspection in the ICU the patient was in moderate respiratory distress. He appeared uncomfortable, and he complained that he could

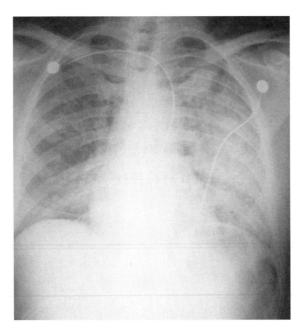

Fig. 21-1

not move very well and that he was becoming short of breath. His blood pressure was 125/78, heart rate was 93 bpm, respiratory rate was 21/min, and core temperature was normal. His skin appeared pale, and when he was asked to cough, he demonstrated an adequate, although nonproductive cough. Upon palpation, tenderness was noted over his anterior chest area, and dull percussion notes were elicited over both lower lung regions. On auscultation, bilateral bronchial breath sounds were heard. His oxygen saturation measured by pulse oximetry (Sp_{O_2}) was 95%, and his ABGs on a 3 L/min oxygen nasal cannula were pH 7.51, Pa_{CO_2} 29 mm Hg, HCO_3^- 22 mmol/L, and Pa_{O_2} 68 mm Hg. His chest x-ray film showed "ground glass" infiltrates throughout both lung fields (Fig. 21-1). The process was more extensive than that noted on admission.

RESPONSE 1

On the basis of the above clinical information, write your SOAP in the following space.

S _____

_____

O _____

_____

_____

_____

_____

_____

A _____

_____

P _____

3 DAYS AFTER SURGERY

At this time the patient paged the nurse and stated he was feeling worse. Respiratory care was called. Upon observation the patient appeared cyanotic. His respiratory rate was 30/min, his blood pressure was 165/95, and his heart rate was 110 bpm. His rectal temperature was 38.8°C (101.8° F). His anterior chest was still tender. Bronchial breath sounds and crackles were heard throughout both lung fields. His Sp_{O_2} was 75%, and his arterial blood gas values were pH 7.56, Pa_{CO_2} 24 mm Hg, HCO_3^- 18 mmol/L, and Pa_{O_2} 35 mm Hg. No recent chest x-ray film was available, but one had been ordered.

RESPONSE 2

On the basis of the above clinical information, write your SOAP in the following space.

S _____

O _____

A _____

P _____

30 MINUTES LATER

The respiratory therapist assigned to monitor and evaluate the patient at this time noted the following: The patient's respiratory rate was 18/min, his blood pressure was 170/97, and his heart rate was 150 bpm. His rectal temperature was 37.8° C (100° F). He was cyanotic, and he no longer responded verbally when asked questions. On auscultation, bronchial breath sounds and crackles could be heard bilaterally. His Sp_{O_2} was 69%, and his arterial blood gas values were pH 7.31, Pa_{CO_2} 48 mm Hg, HCO_3^- 22 mmol/L, Pa_{O_2} 31 mm Hg. A current chest x-ray film showed increased opacities throughout both lung fields.

RESPONSE 3

On the basis of the above clinical information, write your SOAP in the following space.

S _____

O _____

A _____

P

↔ KEY POINT QUESTIONS | *For Adult Respiratory Distress Syndrome (DRG 99/100)*

1. **Basic Concept Formation**
   a. What pulmonary conditions are associated with *trauma?*
   b. What pulmonary conditions are associated with *infection?*
   c. Is ARDS an acute pulmonary illness usually requiring ventilator therapy?

2. **Data Base Formation**
   a. What are the predisposing and *etiologic factors* associated with ARDS?
   b. What is the systemic inflammatory response syndrome (SIRS)?
   c. What is your understanding of the *pathophysiology of ARDS?*
   d. What is your *vision of the pathology* of ARDS?
   e. What should be the *goals of therapy* for such patients?
   f. Which *standard TDPs* would achieve these goals?
   g. List the *expected outcomes, possible adverse effects,* and *monitors* of each protocol you have selected.

3. **Assessment**
   a. Did this patient initially or subsequently demonstrate any of the *clinical manifestations* of ARDS? If so, what were they?
   b. Did this patient have any of the *risk factors* associated with SIRS/ARDS?
   c. Did this patient demonstrate any of the *pathophysiologic alterations* associated with ARDS?
   d. What *specific clinical manifestations* did this patient demonstrate that helped you decide on the *severity* of his condition?
   e. Did the patient demonstrate any of the complications seen in other cases of ARDS?

4. **Application**
   a. Oxygen therapy (was/was not) indicated because _____.
   b. Monitoring (was/was not) indicated because _____.
   c. Hyperinflation therapy (was/was not) indicated because _____.

5. **Evaluation**
   a. What are the expected *results* of each aspect of therapy selected?
   b. How will you *monitor* patient response?
   c. How can you increase or decrease the *intensity* or *frequency* of each modality as needed?
   d. What are the *advantages* and *disadvantages* of each treatment modality?
   e. What if the patient improves?
   f. What if he doesn't?

6. **Boundary Awareness**
   a. How would you know that *this* patient is not improving or getting worse?
   b. When should you ask a supervisor for help?
   c. When should you call the patient's physician?
   d. How would you recognize actual or impending ventilatory failure in this patient?
   e. What *dangers* are there in the treatments you have selected?

22

Idiopathic (infant) Respiratory Distress Syndrome

CASE STUDY

ADMITTING HISTORY

The patient was a 1644 g (3 lb, 10 oz) boy born 8 weeks early (32 weeks' gestation). Of concern to the nurses was the mother's lack of interest in her baby's care. The mother was an unmarried, 17-year-old white high school dropout who planned to put this child up for adoption. Before this admission the mother, whose pregnancy had been considered high risk, was seen for prenatal care only once. At the prenatal visit she was accompanied by her sister, who lived with her in a small mobile home. Shortly after this visit the sister moved to a large nearby town, where she planned to study to become a certified nurse assistant. The mother continued to live in the mobile home with her live-in boy friend, who was out of work. The mother worked as a checkout clerk at a small grocery store.

At this time the mother appeared moderately nervous as she sat up in bed talking to her social worker in preparation for her discharge. The mother looked thin and poorly nourished and constantly requested to go to the smoking room. Because of the mother's obvious disinterest, little progress was made regarding her follow-up, the baby's present condition, or the baby's adoption. In fact, she appeared quite anxious to be discharged, despite its being only 5 hours since the delivery.

PHYSICAL EXAMINATION

In the neonatal intensive care unit the baby was seen to be in mild respiratory distress. The Apgar scores at delivery were 4 and 6. On observation the baby appeared mildly cyanotic and demonstrated intercostal retractions and nasal flaring with all respirations. A mild, gruntlike cry was noted.

The baby's vital signs were respiratory rate 74/min, blood pressure 50/20, and apical heart rate 180 bpm. Auscultation revealed bilateral crackles and sighing breath sounds. A stat chest x-ray film (Fig. 22-1) showed mild haziness and air bronchograms in both lung bases consistent with onset of infant respiratory distress syndrome (IRDS). The infant was placed on an F_{IO_2} of 0.4 via an oxygen hood. Umbilical arterial blood gas values were pH 7.52, $Paco_2$ 29 mm Hg, HCO_3^- 21 mmol/L, and Pao_2 49 mm Hg.

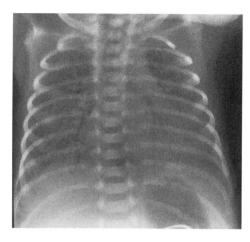

Fig. 22-1

<table>
<tr><td>RESPONSE 1</td></tr>
</table>

On the basis of the above information, write your SOAP in the following space.

S _____

_____

O _____

_____

_____

_____

_____

_____

_____

A _____

_____

_____

_____

_____

_____

_____

P _____

_____

_____

_____

_____

16 HOURS AFTER DELIVERY

At this time the baby was placed on a time-cycled, pressure-limited synchronized intermittent mandatory ventilation (SIMV) rate of 30 breaths per minute, inspiratory time 0.5 seconds, peak inspiratory pressure (PIP) of 20 cm H_2O, an F_{IO_2} of 0.6, and positive end-expiratory pressure (PEEP) of 3 cm H_2O. The baby had no spontaneous breaths. The baby's blood pressure was 60/40, and the apical heart rate was 184 bpm. On auscultation, harsh bronchial breath sounds and fine crackles could be heard bilaterally. A recent chest x-ray film revealed a dense, ground-glass appearance throughout both lung fields. Umbilical arterial blood gas values were pH 7.28, $Paco_2$ 53 mm Hg, HCO_3^- 19 mmol/L, and Pao_2 57 mm Hg.

RESPONSE 2

On the basis of the above information, write your SOAP in the following space.

S _____

O _____

A _____

P _____

48 HOURS LATER

The baby remained intubated and on mechanical ventilation. The ventilator was in the continuous positive airway pressure (CPAP) mode at a pressure setting of 3 cm H_2O, with an F_{IO_2} of 0.45. The infant's vital signs showed a spontaneous respiratory rate of 42/min, a blood pressure of 74/50, and an apical heart rate of 120 bpm. On auscultation, clear, normal vesicular breath sounds were heard. A morning chest x-ray film revealed substantial improvement in the lung fields. Umbilical arterial blood gas values were pH 7.42, Pa_{CO_2} 37 mm Hg, HCO_3^- 24 mmol/L, and Pa_{O_2} 162 mm Hg.

RESPONSE 3

On the basis of the above information, write your SOAP in the following space.

S

O

A

P

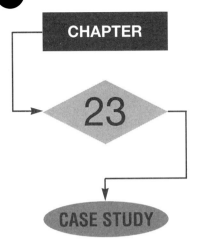

CHAPTER

23

Chronic Interstitial Lung Disease

CASE STUDY

ADMITTING HISTORY

This 56-year-old black woman was seen at the health maintenance organization (HMO) clinic associated with her job because of shortness of breath and an ongoing dry, hacking cough. Before this visit she had seldom seen a physician, as she had always perceived herself to be in perfect health. As a child, she was rarely ill and was only seen for immunizations and preschool physicals.

This woman, a well-known editor at a prestigious publishing house, felt that she had "little time" in her busy life to go through the "hassle" that her HMO required to make an appointment with a physician. Her last experience with the HMO system had been frustrating. She especially did not approve of the physician assigned to see her.

On this day, her worst fears were confirmed. For almost 5 hours she was shuffled from one waiting room to another, filling out forms, giving blood samples, and taking pulmonary function tests (PFT). During this time the closest person to a physician she saw was a young physician's assistant (PA), who slowly took a thorough history. As the PA was closing her interview with the patient, the physician entered the room. The patient sarcastically stated, "You mean, I'm finally going to see a real doctor?"

PHYSICAL EXAMINATION

On observation the patient appeared as a stunning, well-nourished woman who looked much younger than her stated years. Her clothes were impeccable, and her simple but elegant jewelry was "outstanding." The patient stated that she made an appointment because of her recent inability to participate in aerobic exercise classes at work. She said that her shortness of breath, which had progressively worsened over the past several weeks, was accompanied by a dry, hacking cough. She felt her cough was especially annoying. It awakened her from sleep at night. At first, she said, she tried to just cut down on her aerobic classes, but recently she had been unable to tolerate them at all. She claimed never to have smoked.

As she talked, she frequently demonstrated pursed-lip breathing. Her cough was frequent, dry, and nonproductive and was obviously annoying to her. She had a mild-to-moderate degree of digital clubbing, and her nail beds were cyanotic. She also demonstrated a mild degree of peripheral edema, and her neck veins were slightly distended. Her liver was enlarged and tender.

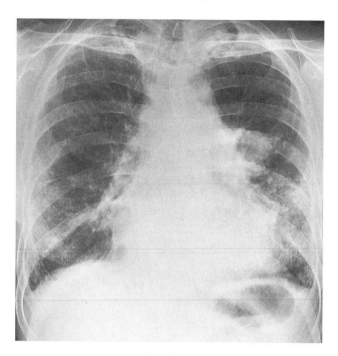

Fig. 23-1

Her vital signs were blood pressure 145/90, heart rate 96 bpm, respiratory rate 28/min, and temperature normal. On auscultation, bronchial breath sounds and crackles could be heard bilaterally. Over the lung bases, tactile, vocal fremitus was notable. Percussion was unremarkable.

Her PFT findings obtained a few hours earlier showed both a restrictive and an obstructive lung disorder, and the pulmonary diffusion capacity of carbon monoxide (D_{LCO}) was 50% of predicted. Her chest x-ray film revealed bilateral diffuse interstitial infiltrates and nodular densities in her lower lung lobes. Air bronchograms were also seen. Her heart was enlarged, suggesting right ventricular hypertrophy (Fig. 23-1). Her laboratory work showed an increase in IgM, IgG, and IgA antibodies. Her arterial blood gases on room air were pH 7.53, Pa_{CO_2} 29 mm Hg, HCO_3^- 21 mmol/L, and Pa_{O_2} 61 mm Hg. At this point the physician elected to admit the patient to the hospital. The physician also requested a respiratory care consultation and scheduled a transbronchial lung biopsy.

RESPONSE 1

On the basis of the above information, write your SOAP in the following space.

S _____

_____

O _____

_____

_____

_____

_____

A _____

P _____

2 DAYS AFTER ADMISSION

The respiratory care practitioner found the patient sitting up in bed editing a manuscript. She quickly complained to the therapist that she had a lot of work to do and that she was getting tired of being in the hospital. Despite her verbal enthusiasm to leave, she appeared weak, fatigued, and in obvious respiratory distress. She still had a frequent, dry cough. She often demonstrated pursed-lip breathing as she talked, and her nail beds were still cyanotic.

Her vital signs were blood pressure 142/91, heart rate 90 bpm, respiratory rate 23/min, and temperature normal. On auscultation, bronchial breath sounds and crackles were heard bilaterally. The histology report regarding the transbronchial lung biopsy established a diagnosis of sarcoidosis.

A morning chest x-ray film showed continued bilateral diffuse interstitial infiltrates and nodular densities in lower lung lobes. Air bronchograms were also seen. A gallium lung scan indicated moderate pulmonary activity. Evidence of cor pulmonale was still present. The patient's peak expiratory flow rate (PEFR) both before and after bronchodilator therapy was 280 L/min. Her arterial blood gas values were pH 7.48, Pa_{CO_2} 32 mm Hg, HCO_3^- 23 mmol/L, and Pa_{O_2} 67 mm Hg. The patient's oxygen saturation measured by pulse oximetry (Sp_{O_2}) was 94%.

RESPONSE 2

On the basis of the above information, write your SOAP in the following space.

S _____

O _____

_____

_____

_____

_____

_____

A _____

_____

_____

_____

_____

_____

_____

P _____

_____

_____

_____

_____

_____

THE NEXT DAY

On this day the physician requested a repeat respiratory care evaluation and recommendations regarding the patient's discharge. The respiratory care practitioner noted that the patient was not in respiratory distress on her present oxygen setting. Although she appeared comfortable, she still had a frequent, dry, hacking cough, and she demonstrated pursed-lip breathing as she talked. She stated she felt much better. Her nail beds no longer appeared cyanotic.

Her vital signs were blood pressure 133/86, heart rate 86 bpm, respiratory rate 15/min, and temperature normal. On auscultation, bronchial breath sounds were heard bilaterally. A morning chest x-ray film showed continued bilateral diffuse interstitial infiltrates and nodular densities. Air bronchograms were also seen. Her arterial blood gas values were pH 7.44, $Paco_2$ 36 mm Hg, HCO_3^- 23 mmol/L, and Pao_2 84 mm Hg. The patient's Spo_2 was 95%.

RESPONSE 3

On the basis of the above information, write your SOAP in the following space.

S _____

_____

O _____

_____
_____
_____
_____
_____

A _____

_____
_____
_____
_____
_____
_____
_____

P _____

_____
_____
_____
_____
_____

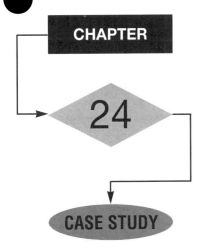

CHAPTER

24

CASE STUDY

Guillain-Barré Syndrome

ADMITTING HISTORY

This 48-year-old career U.S. Navy physician was seen in the hospital base clinic because of an acute onset of severe muscle weakness. He had joined the navy immediately after medical school. Throughout his time in the service he had the opportunity to pursue his passion: competitive water ski jumping. For many years he had been number 1 at most tournaments, including the nationals held yearly. For almost 25 years he progressed through the age divisions, always remaining the top seed, always capturing the highest title.

The patient was in outstanding physical condition. He was an avid runner and weight lifter, and during the off season he would often travel to a warm climate to practice his water ski jumping. He never smoked, and he was never hospitalized. He had an occasional cold, for which he was treated by his peers. About 2 years ago he had begun to focus all his attention on his 19-year-old son, who was quickly following in his footsteps, having just captured the Men's 1 division himself.

The patient claimed to have been well until 2 weeks before his admission, at which time he had a flulike syndrome for 3 days. About 10 days after returning to work, he noticed a tingling sensation in his feet during his morning patient rounds. By dinner time that same day the tingling sensation had radiated from his feet to about the level of his knees. Thinking he was just tired from being on his feet all day, he went to bed early that evening. The next morning, however, his legs were completely numb, although he could still move them. Becoming alarmed, he had his son drive him to the clinic. After examining him, his doctor (a personal friend) admitted him for a diagnostic workup and observation.

Over the next 3 days the laboratory results showed that the patient's cerebrospinal fluid had an elevated protein concentration with a normal cell count. The electrodiagnostic studies showed a progressive ascending paralysis of the patient's arms and legs. The patient began to have difficulty eating and swallowing his food. The respiratory care practitioners, who were monitoring the patient's vital capacity, pulse oximetry, and arterial blood gas values, reported a progressive deterioration in all the values. A diagnosis of Guillain Barré syndrome was made and was written in the patient's chart.

When the patient's arterial blood gas values were pH 7.31, $Paco_2$ 49 mm Hg, HCO_3^- 24 mmol/L, and Pao_2 86 mm Hg (on a 2 L/min O_2 cannula), the respiratory therapist called the doctor and reported the assessment of acute ventilatory failure.

The doctor had the patient transferred to the intensive care unit (ICU), intubated, and placed on a mechanical ventilator. The patient's initial ventilator settings were IMV mode, 12 breaths per minute, tidal volume 0.85 L, and F_{IO_2} 0.40.

Fifteen minutes after the patient was committed to the ventilator, he appeared comfortable. No spontaneous breaths were noted in between the 12 intermittent mandatory ventilations. His vital signs were blood pressure 126/82 and heart rate 68 bpm. A chest x-ray film taken by portable machine revealed that the endotracheal tube was in a good position and that the lungs were adequately aerated. Normal vesicular breath sounds were auscultated over both lung fields. His arterial blood gas values were pH 7.51, Pa_{CO_2} 29 mm Hg, HCO_3^- 22 mmol/L, Pa_{O_2} 204 mm Hg. His oxygen saturation measured by pulse oximetry (Sp_{O_2}) was 98%.

RESPONSE 1

On the basis of the above information, write your SOAP in the following space.

S _____

O _____

A _____

P _____

3 DAYS AFTER ADMISSION

The patient's cardiopulmonary status up to this time was unremarkable. No improvement was seen in his muscular paralysis. No changes had been made in his ventilator settings over the past 48 hours. His skin color was good. Palpation and percussion of the chest were unremarkable. On auscultation, however, crackles and rhonchi could be heard over both lung fields.

Moderate amounts of white, clear secretions were being suctioned from the patient's endotracheal tube on a regular basis. His vital signs were blood pressure 124/83, heart rate 74 bpm, and rectal temperature 37.7° C (99.8°F). A recent chest x-ray film taken by portable machine revealed no significant pathology. His arterial blood gas values were pH 7.44, $Paco_2$ 35 mm Hg, HCO_3^- 24 mmol/L, and Pao_2 98 mm Hg. His Spo_2 was 97%.

RESPONSE 2

On the basis of the above information, write your SOAP in the following space.

S _____

O _____

_____

_____

_____

_____

_____

A _____

_____

_____

_____

_____

_____

_____

P _____

_____

_____

_____

_____

_____

5 DAYS AFTER ADMISSION

The patient's muscular paralysis remained unchanged. The patient's skin color was good, and no remarkable information was found during palpation and percussion. Although crackles and rhonchi could still be heard over both lung fields, they were not so intense as they had been 48 hours before. A small amount of clear secretions was suctioned out of the patient's endotracheal tube. His vital signs were blood pressure 118/79, heart rate 68 bpm, and temperature normal. A recent chest x-ray film taken by portable machine was reported as normal. His arterial blood gas values were pH 7.42, $Paco_2$ 37 mm Hg, HCO_3^- 24 mmol/L, and Pao_2 97 mm Hg. His Spo_2 was 97%.

RESPONSE 3

On the basis of the above information, write your SOAP in the following space.

S _____

_____

O _____

_____

_____

_____

_____

_____

A _____

_____

_____

_____

_____

_____

_____

P _____

_____

_____

_____

_____

_____

25 Myasthenia Gravis

ADMITTING HISTORY

This 35-year-old Spanish American woman was a school teacher with a 3-year-old son and an unemployed husband, who was still "finding his real place in life." The patient was a high achiever. Recently she had received her Ph.D. in education, but continued to work in the classroom with the grade school children she loved so much, and had been named teacher of the year in the large city where she lived. Her colleagues at school considered her a nonstop worker. She had never smoked.

At home she was always on the move. She had just finished remodeling her kitchen and two bathrooms. She also did her own backyard landscaping on the weekends, a job she particularly enjoyed. She read and played with her son whenever they could have time together. Although she enjoyed cooking (a skill she had learned from her mother), she did not like to grocery shop. Fortunately this was a chore that her husband enjoyed doing.

Three weeks before the current admission the patient noticed that her eyes "felt tired." She began to experience slight double vision. Thinking that she had just been working too hard, she slowed down a bit and went to bed earlier for about a week. However, she progressively felt weaker. Her legs quickly became tired, and she began having trouble chewing her food. Concerned, the patient finally went to see her doctor. After reviewing the patient's recent history and performing a careful physical examination, the physician admitted her to the hospital for further evaluation and treatment.

Over the next 48 hours the patient's physical status progressively declined. After the administration of edrophonium (Tensilon) there was a significant increase in her muscle function that lasted about 10 minutes. Electromyography disclosed extensive muscle involvement and a high degree of fatigability in all the affected muscles. A diagnosis of myasthenia gravis was made and noted in the patient's chart.

The patient began to choke and aspirate food during meals, and a nasogastric feeding tube was inserted. Her speech became more and more slurred. Her upper eyelids drooped, and she was unable to hold her head up off her pillow when requested to do so. The respiratory therapists who monitored her vital capacity, pulse oximetry, and arterial blood gas values reported a progressive worsening in all the parameters monitored.

When the patient's arterial blood gas values were pH 7.35, Pa_{CO_2} 45 mm Hg, HCO_3^- 24 mmol/L, and Pa_{O_2} 69 mm Hg (on room air), the respiratory therapist called the physician and reported his assessment of impending ventilatory failure. The doctor had the patient transferred to the intensive care unit, intubated, and placed on a mechanical ventilator. The patient's initial ventilator settings were IMV 10 breaths per minute, tidal volume 0.8 L, and F_{IO_2} 0.5.

Twenty-five minutes after the patient was placed on the ventilator, she appeared stable. No spontaneous ventilations were seen. Her vital signs were blood pressure 132/86 and heart rate 90 bpm. A chest x-ray film taken by portable machine had been ordered but had not yet been taken. Normal bronchial vesicular breath sounds were auscultated over the right lung, and diminished-to-absent breath sounds were auscultated over the patient's left lung. On an F_{IO_2} of 0.5, her arterial blood gas values were pH 7.28, Pa_{CO_2} 58 mm Hg, HCO_3^- 24 mmol/L, and Pa_{O_2} 52 mm Hg. Her oxygen saturation measured by pulse oximetry (Sp_{O_2}) was 80%.

RESPONSE 1

On the basis of the above information, write your SOAP in the following space.

S _____

O _____

A _____

P _____

45 MINUTES LATER

After the patient's endotracheal tube was pulled back 4 cm, normal vesicular breath sounds could be auscultated over the left lung. The chest x-ray film confirmed that the endotracheal tube was in a good position above the carina and that both lungs were adequately aerated.

Her vital signs were blood pressure 123/75, heart rate 74 bpm, and temperature normal. The ventilator settings were readjusted, and repeat arterial blood gases were pH 7.53, $Paco_2$ 27 mm Hg, HCO_3^- 22 mmol/L, and Pao_2 176 mm Hg. Her Spo_2 was 98%.

RESPONSE 2

On the basis of the above information, write your SOAP in the following space.

S _____

_____

O _____

_____

_____

_____

_____

_____

_____

A _____

_____

_____

_____

_____

_____

_____

P _____

_____

_____

_____

_____

_____

_____

3 DAYS AFTER ADMISSION

No changes had to be made in the patient's ventilator settings over the previous 48 hours. No improvement was seen in her muscular paralysis. The patient appeared pale, and her vital signs were blood pressure 146/88, heart rate 92 bpm, and temperature 37.9° C (100.2° F). Large amounts of thick, yellowish sputum were being suctioned from the patient's endotracheal tube every 30 minutes or so.

Rhonchi were auscultated over both lung fields. A sputum sample was obtained and sent to the laboratory to be cultured. A recent chest x-ray film taken by portable machine showed a new infiltrate in the right lower lobe consistent with pneumonia or atelectasis. The patient's arterial blood gas values were pH 7.28, $Paco_2$ 36 mm Hg, HCO_3^- 17 mmol/L, Pao_2 41 mm Hg. Her Spo_2 was 69%.

RESPONSE 3

On the basis of the above information, write your SOAP in the following space.

S _____

O _____

A _____

P _____

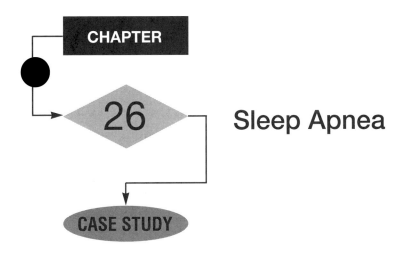

CHAPTER

26 Sleep Apnea

CASE STUDY

ADMITTING HISTORY

This 55-year-old white man had been in the U.S. Marine Corp for over 25 years when he retired with honors at the age of 46 with the rank of sergeant. He had done tours in Vietnam, Grenada, and Beirut. His last assignment was in Iraq and Kuwait during Operation Desert Storm. During his military career he had received several medals, including a Purple Heart for a leg wound received in Vietnam while he was pulling a fellow marine to safety. During his last 3 years in the service he was assigned to a desk job, working with new recruits as they progressed through various stages of boot camp.

Although it was not mandatory that he retire, he felt it was time to do so. He had gained a great deal of weight over the years, and his ability to meet the physical challenge of being a marine had become progressively more difficult. In addition, when he was doing paper work at his office, he was aware of the fact that he was catnapping while on the job. He knew that if he had observed a fellow marine sleeping on the job, he would have been quick to issue a severe reprimand. In view of these developments the patient regretfully retired from the service.

For a few years after he retired he continued to work for the marines as a retired volunteer at a local recruitment office. At first he enjoyed this job a great deal. He often found that his past military experiences enhanced his ability to talk to new recruits. Over the past few years, however, he found it more and more difficult to work in the recruiting office. His attendance had become increasingly more sporadic. He was often tardy for work. He told the other recruitment volunteers that he was always tired and that he was having severe morning headaches. His coworkers frequently found him to be irritable and quick to anger.

The patient was having trouble at home too. Several months before this admission his wife had started sleeping in a room vacated by their daughter who had recently married. She claimed she could no longer sleep with her husband because of his loud snoring and constant thrashing about in bed. About this time the patient became clinically depressed and sexually impotent. Despite much discussion and encouragement from his wife to do so, the patient did not seek medical advice until he became extremely short of breath a few hours before this admission. His wife drove him to the local emergency room, where he was evaluated.

PHYSICAL EXAMINATION

Upon observation the patient appeared in severe respiratory distress. He was obese, weighing over 160 kg (355 lb), and perspiring profusely. His skin was cyanotic, and his neck veins were distended. He had 4+ edema of his feet and ankles extending to midcalf. His blood pressure was 194/118; his heart rate was 78 bpm; his respiratory rate was 22/min; and his temperature was normal. Although the patient was in obvious discomfort, he stated that he was breathing okay. His wife quickly piped up with "There's that damn marine coming out again."

The patient's breath sounds were normal but diminished. It was believed that the diminished breath sounds were primarily due to the patient's obesity. Palpation was unremarkable, and percussion was unreliable because of the patient's obesity. A chest x-ray film showed cardiomegaly; the lungs appeared normal. To treat presumed cor pulmonale, the physician immediately started the patient on digitalis and diuretics. His arterial blood gas values on room air were pH 7.54, Pa_{CO_2} 58 mm Hg, HCO_3^- 39 mmol/L, and Pa_{O_2} 52 mm Hg. His oxygen saturation measured by pulse oximetry (Sp_{O_2}) was 87%.

Because of the patient's history and present clinical manifestations, the respiratory therapist on duty suspected that the patient had obstructive sleep apnea. The therapist suggested this to the emergency room physician, who requested a polysomnographic sleep study. The physician agreed and asked the respiratory therapist to document her assessment.

RESPONSE 1

On the basis of the above information, write your SOAP in the following space.

S _____

O _____

A _____

P _____

OVER THE NEXT 72 HOURS

The diagnosis of severe obstructive sleep apnea was quickly established. Along with the patient's classic history of obstructive sleep apnea, a polysomnographic sleep study documented over 325 periods of obstructive apnea. In addition to the fact that the patient had a short, muscular neck and was extremely overweight, an oropharyngeal examination revealed a small mouth and large tongue for body size. The free margin of the soft palate hung low in the oropharynx, nearly obliterating the view behind it. The uvula was 4+ widened and elongated; the tonsillar pillars were 3+ widened. Air entry through the nares was reduced bilaterally. A laboratory report showed the patient's hematocrit to be 51% and hemoglobin to be 17g/dl.

A complete pulmonary function study (PFT) showed that the patient had a severe restrictive disorder. In addition, a sawtooth pattern was seen in the maximal inspiratory and expiratory flow-volume loops. A chest x-ray film obtained on the patient's second day of hospitalization showed reduction in the patient's heart size, and the lung parenchyma were clear. The patient stated that he was breathing much better.

Upon inspection the patient no longer appeared short of breath. Although he still appeared flushed, he did not look as cyanotic as he had when he was first admitted. His neck veins were no longer distended, and the peripheral edema of his ankles and feet had improved. His breath sounds were clear but diminished. His arterial blood gas values were pH 7.38, $Paco_2$ 82 mm Hg, HCO_3^- 44 mmol/L, and Pao_2 66 mm Hg. His Spo_2 was 91%. The physician again called for a respiratory care consultation.

RESPONSE 2

On the basis of the above information, write your SOAP in the following space.

S _____

_____

O _____

_____

_____

_____

_____

_____

_____

A _____

_____

_____

_____

_____

_____

_____

_____

P

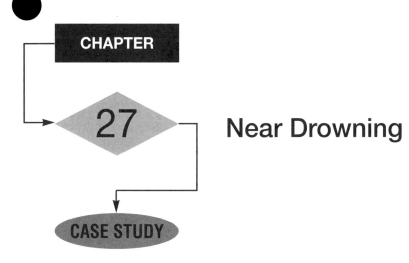

CHAPTER

27 Near Drowning

CASE STUDY

ADMITTING HISTORY

This 18-year-old white boy was part of a 300-student graduating class from a Colorado high school in the foothills of the Rocky Mountains. Graduation took place in late May. The day before their graduation ceremony about 80 students spent most of the day and evening in the mountains roasting a pig, playing volleyball, and consuming large quantities of beer. It was later reported that there were seven empty kegs of beer tied down in one pickup truck alone.

Driving down the narrow and curving mountain road was difficult to do sober during the daylight hours, let alone at night with an elevated blood alcohol level. Unfortunately the patient, who was intoxicated, chose to drive his pickup home. His girlfriend and his best friend were passengers in the vehicle. Several other cars and trucks filled with students also were traveling down the mountain at the same time. About 10 miles out of town the patient's truck suddenly swerved off the road, went down a 7.5 m (25 ft) embankment, and plunged into a river. Within seconds the truck was completely submerged. It was later reported that the water temperature was about 13° C (55° F).

The patient's girlfriend and best friend swam to safety. The patient did not. The patient was not breathing when he was pulled from the wreckage by three students from the truck following his. It was later estimated that the patient was trapped underneath the water for about 10 minutes. Cardiopulmonary resuscitation (CPR) was administered by two students who recently had completed a first aid course. Another student who had a cellular phone called 911.

When the paramedics arrived, the patient was not conscious, and his pupils were fixed and dilated. He had a pulse but no respirations. An oral airway was inserted, and the patient was manually ventilated with 100% oxygen attached to an E-tank. En route to the hospital the patient's wet clothing was removed, and he was wrapped in several warm blankets. The patient's vital signs were blood pressure 126/84, heart rate 118 bpm, respiratory rate 26/min, and temperature 31° C (88.7° F). His oxygen saturation measured by pulse oximetry (Spo$_2$) was 91%.

Upon arrival in the emergency department the patient was no longer being manually ventilated by the paramedics. The patient demonstrated a rapid, gaspinglike breathing pattern. He was semiconscious and thrashing around. Despite the fact that the patient was on a nonrebreathing mask, his skin was cyanotic. His pupils were no longer fixed and dilated. Except for some minor bruises and abrasions, no traumatic injuries were apparent.

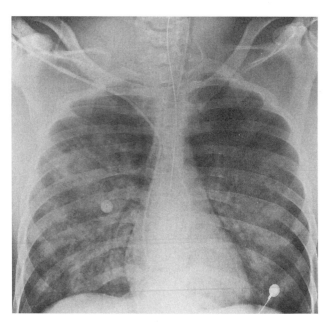

Fig. 27-1

His vital signs were blood pressure 137/89, heart rate 122 bpm, respiratory rate 28/min, and rectal temperature 32.3° C (90.3° F). Palpation of the chest was nonremarkable. Over the lung bases, dull percussion notes were elicited, and fine crackles were auscultated. His arterial blood gas values were pH 7.11, $Paco_2$ 72 mm Hg, HCO_3^- 18 mmol/L, Pao_2 36 mm Hg. The patient's Spo_2 was 57%. Near drowning was written as the diagnosis in the patient's chart.

The patient was intubated, transferred to the intensive care unit, and placed on a mechanical ventilator. His initial ventilator settings were assist/control mode, 12 breaths per minute, tidal volume 750 ml, and F_{IO_2} 0.50. A chest x-ray film taken with a portable machine showed the endotracheal tube was positioned correctly, and bilateral patchy infiltrates were noted in both lower lobes (Fig. 27-1). Twelve minutes after the patient was placed on the ventilator, his arterial blood gas values were pH 7.23, $Paco_2$ 51 mm Hg, HCO_3^- 19 mmol/L, and Pao_2 54 mm Hg. His Spo_2 was 84%.

RESPONSE 1

On the basis of the above information, write your SOAP in the following space.

S _____

_____

O _____

_____

_____

_____

_____

_____

_____

A _____
_____
_____
_____
_____
_____
_____
_____
_____

P _____
_____
_____
_____
_____
_____
_____

45 MINUTES LATER

The patient was sedated and quiet. An arterial catheter and intravenous line were in place. His vital signs were blood pressure 125/86, heart rate 130 bpm, and rectal temperature 33.4° C (92.3° F). The patient's chest assessment data had deteriorated since admission: dull percussion notes were now elicited throughout both lung fields, and more prominent crackles and rhonchi were heard over both lungs. A moderate amount of frothy, white sputum was being suctioned out of the patient's endotracheal tube. Since a recent chest x-ray film was not available, a stat chest x-ray film was ordered by the head nurse. His arterial blood gas values were pH 7.53, Pa_{CO_2} 28 mm Hg, HCO_3^- 21 mmol/L, and Pa_{O_2} 56 mm Hg. His Sp_{O_2} was 89%.

RESPONSE 2

On the basis of the above information, write your SOAP in the following space.

S _____
_____

O _____
_____
_____
_____
_____
_____
_____

A _____

_____

_____

_____

_____

_____

_____

P _____

_____

_____

_____

_____

_____

_____

10 HOURS LATER

The patient's cardiopulmonary status remained critical. The patient was still heavily sedated. His skin was cool and cyanotic. His vital signs were blood pressure 100/60, heart rate 150 bpm, and rectal temperature 39.5° C (103° F). Despite aggressive suctioning and anterior chest percussion and drainage, crackles and rhonchi were now abundant throughout all lung fields. Frothy, pink secretions were difficult to keep out of the patient's endotracheal tube.

Large dosages of diuretics and cardiac agents had been used for some time now but with marginal results. The patient's pupils were again fixed and dilated. A neurologist had been called in for consultation. A recent chest x-ray film taken by portable machine revealed fluffy infiltrate throughout both lung fields that was consistent with a pulmonary edema pattern. His arterial blood gas values were pH 7.35, $Paco_2$ 37 mm Hg, HCO_3^- 23 mmol/L, and Pao_2 47 mm Hg. His Spo_2 was 80%.

RESPONSE 3

On the basis of the above information, write your SOAP in the following space.

S _____

_____

O _____

_____

_____

_____

_____

_____

A _____

_____

_____

_____

_____

_____

_____

P _____

_____

_____

_____

_____

_____

_____

_____

28 Smoke Inhalation and Thermal Injuries

ADMITTING HISTORY

This 46-year-old white man was rescued by the fire department from his two-story home. A taxi cab driver driving by the patient's home at about 4 o'clock in the morning saw the patient's house engulfed with fire and smoke. He reported the fire to his dispatcher, who in turn called the fire department. The fire department arrived about 25 minutes later. Neighbors reported that a single man lived in the house. Five minutes later a fireman exited the house carrying a middle-aged man. The patient had been found in bed unconscious in a smoke- and flame-filled room.

The patient displayed agonal respirations. The patient's left leg, left arm, and anterior trunk were severely burned. No burns were noted on his head or neck. The paramedics immediately inserted an oral airway and started to manually ventilate the patient with 100% oxygen. A pulse was palpable, and the patient was quickly transferred to the ambulance. En route to the hospital an intravenous infusion of Ringer's lactate solution was started, an ampule of bicarbonate was administered, and the remainder of the patient's pajamas was cut away.

The patient was unresponsive to deep pain. His pupils were dilated, and both reacted slowly to intense light. His nasal hairs were singed, and he had a frequent, loose-sounding cough. After each coughing episode the paramedics suctioned a small amount of coal-colored sputum from his oral and nasal pharynx. His vital signs en route to the hospital were blood pressure 153/98 and heart rate 109 bpm. His Spo_2 was 97%.

Upon arrival in the emergency room the patient was immediately intubated and placed on mechanical ventilation. Most of his burns were classified as second degree. His left foot had third-degree burns. After the burns were treated, the patient was transferred to the intensive care unit. The initial ventilator settings were assist/control mode, 14 breaths per minute, tidal volume 800 ml, +5 continuous positive airway pressure (CPAP), and F_{IO_2} 1.0.

Twenty minutes after the patient was placed on the mechanical ventilator, his blood pressure was 157/105 and his heart rate was 112 bpm. There were no spontaneous ventilations. His skin was cherry red. Frothy, sooty appearing sputum was suctioned from the patient's endotracheal tube. Crackles and rhonchi were auscultated over both lung fields. A chest x-ray film taken by portable machine revealed bilateral pulmonary infiltrates consistent with pulmonary edema (Fig. 28-1). The patient's arterial blood gas values were pH 7.52, $Paco_2$ 28 mm Hg, HCO_3^- 22 mmol/L, and Pao_2 202 mm Hg. His oxygen saturation measured by pulse oximetry (Spo_2) was 98%. His COHb was 30%. No cyanide was found in the patient's blood.

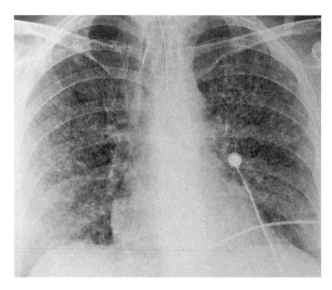

Fig. 28-1

On the basis of the above information, write your SOAP in the following space.

S _____

_____

O _____

_____

_____

_____

_____

_____

_____

A _____

_____

_____

_____

_____

_____

_____

_____

P _____

_____

_____

_____

_____

_____

_____

_____

24 HOURS AFTER ADMISSION

The patient was still unconscious, and his cardiopulmonary status was described as unstable. His COHb was 20% following his first hyperbaric oxygen (HBO) treatment. A pulmonary arterial catheter and central venous pressure line had been inserted. The patient's blood pressure was 127/88, and his heart rate was 82. His total respiratory rate (on assist/control ventilation) was 30/min. All other hemodynamic indices were normal. His skin was still cherry red, and frothy, sooty secretions were still being suctioned from the patient's endotracheal tube every 15 or 20 minutes.

Crackles and rhonchi were still auscultated over both lung fields. A recent chest x-ray film taken by portable machine showed that the endotracheal tube was in a good position and that the pulmonary infiltrates were becoming worse. The patient's arterial blood gas values were pH 7.29, Pa_{CO_2} 37 mm Hg, HCO_3^- 18 mmol/L, and Pa_{O_2} 63 mm Hg.

RESPONSE 2

On the basis of the above information, write your SOAP in the following space.

S _____

_____

O _____

_____

_____

_____

_____

_____

_____

A _____

_____

_____

_____

_____

_____

_____

_____

P _____

_____

_____

_____

_____

_____

_____

4 DAYS AFTER ADMISSION

The patient was conscious but sedated, and his thermal burns were starting to heal nicely; there were no signs of infection. His cardiopulmonary status, however, continued to be unstable. He remained intubated and on assist/control ventilation. Excessive thick, gray and yellow secretions were being suctioned from the patient's endotracheal tube. A sputum culture was positive for *Pseudomonas.*

A recent chest x-ray film showed greater opacity throughout both lung fields, which suggested severe pulmonary edema and atelectasis. In addition, the radiologist also believed the patient was developing ARDS. Shortly after the radiologist's report was received, the respiratory therapist assisted the physician in a therapeutic bronchoscopy. Numerous eschars and mucus plugs were suctioned from the patient's tracheobronchial tree.

The patient's skin was no longer red. A few hours earlier his hemodynamic indices indicated a moderate increase in his pulmonary vascular resistance (PVR) and systemic vascular resistance (SVR) and a moderate decrease in all other parameters. Fluid resuscitation was administered, and all the hemodynamic indices returned to normal. His arterial blood gas values were pH 7.25, Pa_{CO_2} 39 mm Hg, HCO_3^- 18 mmol/L, and Pa_{O_2} 37 mm Hg. Following his second HBO treatment his COHb was 10%. The physician prescribed a repeat hyperbaric treatment despite the fact that the COHb was 10%, since the Pa_{O_2} was so low.

RESPONSE 3

On the basis of the above information, write your SOAP in the following space.

S _____

_____

O _____

_____

_____

_____

_____

_____

A _____

_____

_____

_____

_____

P

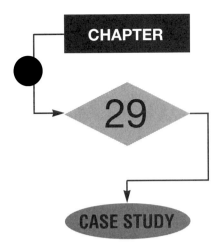

Postoperative Atelectasis

ADMITTING HISTORY

This 43-year-old woman was admitted to the hospital for an exploratory thoracotomy for diagnosis of a 1.5 cm pulmonary nodule that had resisted diagnosis by bronchoscopy and percutaneous needle biopsy. She had been a registered nurse for the past 15 years and up until about a year ago was the director of nursing at this hospital. For the past 4 months she had been working on the night shift as a general floor nurse in a nursing home owned by the hospital. Although she had been considered by most to be an attractive woman, her general appearance over the last several years had progressively declined. For the past 3 years she had rapidly moved from a normal, healthy weight to obesity.

Over the last 6 months she almost always had been seen wearing one of the same three outfits, had quit wearing makeup, and had increased her smoking habit from one to two and a half packs of cigarettes a day. Her general hygiene was poor, and her hair often appeared dirty. Her estranged husband reported that she had been depressed for the past year or so. He described how he had unsuccessfully suggested that they both see a marriage counselor. Frustrated, he moved into his brother's apartment a few miles away from his wife. Despite these events, they continued to speak to each other on a regular basis.

The patient had been seen in the preoperative education area before her surgery. Her forced vital capacity (FVC) was normal, but her forced expiratory volume in 1 second (FEV_1) was 50% of predicted. She frequently generated a spontaneous, strong cough, producing moderate amounts of yellow sputum. She was instructed on the use of bronchodilator therapy via metered dose inhaler (MDI) and deep breathing and coughing (DB&C) techniques. Her attention span, however, was poor, and she continually sang words of praise and recognition to every employee who passed by her room. She also flooded the respiratory therapist with "aren't you wonderful" phrases as the therapist tried to have her demonstrate the various techniques she would be required to perform after her surgery.

In the postanesthesia area, however, she continually used foul language and threatened to have everyone fired. Her physician ordered a sedative and then had her transferred to the postoperative unit. Over the next 2 hours the patient's general respiratory status declined. Concerned, the patient's primary nurse paged the physician. Busy in another part of the hospital, the physician requested a respiratory care consult.

PHYSICAL EXAMINATION (Time: 1330)

The respiratory care practitioner noted the patient was awake and in obvious respiratory distress. Her vital signs were blood pressure 185/140, heart rate 130 bpm, respiratory rate 35/min, and temperature normal. She demonstrated tachypnea and a frequent spontaneous, weak cough. A moderate amount of yellow sputum was often expectorated during a coughing episode. She appeared cyanotic and quickly stated, "Damn, my gut really hurts, . . . and I can't seem to get any air."

Over the left lower lung region, diminished breath sounds were noted. Bronchial breath sounds and dull percussion notes were noted over the right lower lung region. The nurse indicated that the patient's incentive spirometry (IS) volume was only about 40% of her preoperative value when she could get the patient to attempt to use the device. Her oxygen saturation measured by pulse oximetry (Sp_{O_2}) on a 2 L/min oxygen cannula was 77%. Arterial blood gases obtained by the respiratory care practitioner were pH 7.57, Pa_{CO_2} 23 mm Hg, HCO_3^- 21 mmol/L, and Pa_{O_2} 43 mm Hg. No recent chest x-ray film was available. As the therapist documented the above data, the patient's physician entered the room and stated, "I'll do anything to keep this patient off the ventilator. Keep me informed." She then prescribed some medication for the patient's pain and quickly left the room.

RESPONSE 1

On the basis of the above information, write your SOAP in the following space.

S _____

O _____

A _____

P _____

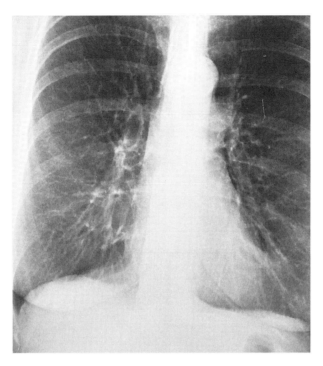

Fig. 29-1

DAY 1 AFTER SURGERY

Despite the fact that the patient needed aggressive respiratory care, she was generally uncooperative or unwilling to tolerate various treatment modalities. At this point her skin was blue, cool, and damp. Her eyes were closed, and she was unresponsive to questions. She still demonstrated a weak cough every few minutes. Although sputum retention was suspected, none was actually seen. It was believed that the patient was swallowing any sputum produced. Her vital signs were blood pressure 188/144, heart rate 135 bpm, respiratory rate 36/min, and rectal temperature 38.1° C (100.6° F).

Chest assessment found dull percussion notes, bronchial breath sounds, and crackles over the right middle and both lower lobes. A chest x-ray film taken by portable machine revealed that she had atelectasis in the right middle and both lower lobes. Air bronchograms were also noted in this area (Fig. 29-1). Her Spo_2 was 72%. Her arterial blood gas values were pH 7.55, $Paco_2$ 29 mm Hg, HCO_3^- 22 mmol/L, and Pao_2 46 mm Hg.

RESPONSE 2

On the basis of the above information, write your SOAP in the following space.

S _____

_____

O _____

_____

_____

_____

_____

A _____

_____

_____

_____

_____

_____

_____

_____

P _____

_____

_____

_____

_____

_____

7 HOURS LATER

The respiratory care practitioner working on the pulmonary consult team at this time found the patient in obvious respiratory distress. Her skin was cyanotic, cool, and damp. The patient stated, "I think I'm dying." No cough was observed at this time. No right-sided chest excursion could be seen, and her trachea was deviated to the right.

Her vital signs were blood pressure 192/148, heart rate 142 bpm, and respiratory rate 20/min. Bronchial breath sounds, crackles, and dull percussion notes were found over the right middle and lower lobes. Dull percussion notes and no breath sounds were noted over left lower lobe. Her Spo_2 was 62%. Her arterial blood gas values were pH 7.26, $Paco_2$ 53 mm Hg, HCO_3^- 22 mmol/L, and Pao_2 37 mm Hg.

RESPONSE 3

On the basis of the above information, write your SOAP in the following space.

S _____

_____

O _____

_____

_____

_____

_____

_____

A

P

➡ KEY POINT QUESTIONS *For Postoperative Atelectasis (DRG 101/102)*

---

1. **Basic Concept Formation**
   a. What should happen to the volume of an alveolus, lobule, or lobe of the lung if it becomes *airless?*
   b. What would be the effect on oxygenation of pulmonary capillary blood passing such an area?
   c. Name *two simple causes* for atelectasis.
   d. Would coughing, deep breathing, and secretion removal *reverse* some of this pathology?

2. **Data Base Formation**
   a. What is your *vision of the pathology* of pulmonary atelectasis?
   b. What *pathophysiologic mechanisms* are activated as a result of these anatomic alterations?
   c. Are any portions of the *airway model* (Fig. 1-3) abnormal in usual cases of atelectasis?
   d. What changes might be expected if atelectasis is left untreated or allowed to *worsen?*
   e. What are the most common *causes* of atelectasis?
   f. What are the *goals of therapy* for such patients?
   g. Which *standard TDPs* should achieve these purposes?
      (1) List the potential *adverse effects* of each protocol you have selected.
      (2) How would you *monitor* the beneficial or adverse effects of the therapies you have selected?

3. **Assessment**
   a. Did this patient's history suggest that she might develop atelectasis?
   b. Did this patient initially or subsequently demonstrate any evidence of the *clinical manifestations* of atelectasis? If so, what were they?
   c. Did this patient initially demonstrate any evidence of the *pathophysiologic alterations* commonly associated with atelectasis?
   d. What specific clinical manifestations did this patient demonstrate that helped you decide on the *severity* of her condition?

4. **Application**
   a. *Sputum induction* (was/was not) indicated because _____.
   b. *Oxygen therapy* (was/was not) indicated because _____.
   c. *Bronchial hygiene therapy* (was/was not) indicated because _____.
   d. *Hyperinflation therapy* (was/was not) indicated because _____.
   e. *Mechanical ventilation* (was/was not) indicated at some point because _____.
   f. *Pulmonary rehabilitation* (was/was not) indicated because _____.

5. **Evaluation**
   a. What are the expected results of each therapy you have selected? Are there complications from these modalities?
   b. How will you monitor the patient's response to each modality?
   c. How can you up-regulate the intensity and/or the frequency of each modality as needed?
   d. What are the advantages and disadvantages of each treatment modality that you have selected?
   e. What if the patient improves?
   f. What if she doesn't?

6. **Boundary Awareness**
   a. How would you know that *this* patient is not improving or getting worse?
   b. When should you ask a supervisor for help?
   c. When should you call the patient's physician?

APPENDIX I
SUGGESTED SOAP RESPONSES, CASE DISCUSSIONS,
AND KEY POINT ANSWERS

The SOAP responses presented throughout Appendix I are intended only as a guide. Depending on the specific case and severity of the clinical manifestations, other assessments and treatment selections could be appropriate. It also should be noted here that the clinical manifestations in the parentheses to the right of each assessment likely would not appear in the patient's chart. They are presented here only to justify each assessment.

CHAPTER 2 Chronic Bronchitis

RESPONSE 1

S: "I'm unable to breathe. I can't inhale deep enough to cough up secretions, and my stomach is upset."

O: Vitals: HR 125, BP 190/115, RR 30, T 37° C (98.6° F). Barrel chest, labored breathing, use of accessory muscles, digital clubbing, cyanosis, and 1+ pitting ankle edema. Copious thick, yellow sputum. Chest hyperresonant, with rhonchi heard bilaterally. CXR: lungs clear, air trapping, and depressed diaphragm. Hct 58%. HbCO 6%. ABGs (room air): pH 7.53, Pa_{CO_2} 56, HCO_3^- 33, and Pa_{O_2} 43.

A:
- Acute exacerbation of chronic bronchitis (general presentation, sputum, vital signs, ABGs)
- Increased work of breathing (increased heart rate, blood pressure, and respiratory rate)
- Excessive airway secretions (sputum, rhonchi)
  - Infection is likely (thick, yellow secretions)
- Poor ability to mobilize secretions (weak cough)
- Acute alveolar hyperventilation on top of chronic ventilatory failure (ABGs and history)
  - Possible impending ventilatory failure

P: Oxygen therapy per protocol (e.g., use Venturi mask). Bronchial hygiene therapy per protocol (sputum culture). Contact physician regarding possible impending ventilatory failure. Mechanical ventilator on standby. Monitor and reevaluate (e.g., vital signs, ABGs, Sp_{O_2}).

RESPONSE 2

S: "I'm having a bad period."

O: Vitals: HR 130, BP 185/135, RR 28, T 37° C (98.6° F). Use of accessory muscles and pursed-lip breathing. Cough weak and productive of large amounts of thick, yellow sputum. Bilateral rhonchi. ABGs: pH 7.55, Pa_{CO_2} 53, HCO_3^- 32, Pa_{O_2} 41. Sp_{O_2}: 83%.

A:
- Continued acute exacerbation of chronic bronchitis with no improvement over the past 9 hours (general appearance and clinical data)
- Continued increased work of breathing (general appearance, elevated heart rate, blood pressure, and respiratory rate)
- Persistent, excessive airway secretions (sputum, rhonchi)
  - Infection is likely (yellow sputum)
- Poor ability to mobilize secretions (weak cough)
- Acute alveolar hyperventilation on top of chronic ventilatory failure (ABGs and history)
  - Impending ventilatory failure

P: Up-regulate oxygen therapy per protocol. Up-regulate bronchial hygiene therapy per protocol. Contact physican regarding possible impending ventilatory failure. Monitor and reevaluate.

RESPONSE 3

S: "I'm feeling worse again."

O: Vital signs: BP 150/95, HR 140, RR 25 and shallow. Using accessory muscles of respiration and pursed-lip breathing. Cough weak and no sputum production. Expiration is prolonged. Bilateral rhonchi. ABGs: pH 7.28, Pa_{CO_2} 105, HCO_3^- 41, Pa_{O_2} 44, HbCO 2.5%.

A: • Continued exacerbation of chronic bronchitis; unimproved since last evaluation 12 hours ago (general appearance and clinical data)
  • Excessive airway secretions (rhonchi)
  • Poor ability to mobilize secretions (weak cough)
  • Acute ventilatory failure on top of chronic ventilatory failure (ABGs and history)

P: Contact physician stat. Transfer to intensive care unit (ICU) and prepare for intubation and mechanical ventilation. Up-regulate oxygen therapy per protocol. Up-regulate bronchial hygiene therapy per protocol. Monitor and reevaluate after implementation of mechanical ventilation. Repeat CXR after intubation.

Discussion

The return to hospital of a patient with chronic bronchitis who is known not to have complied with therapy in the past is all too familiar to the respiratory care practitioner and his physicians. This patient has persisted in his cigarette smoking habit, refused an attempt at pulmonary rehabilitation, and now has allowed his personal hygiene to deteriorate.

It would be easy to shrug all this off and to discharge him from the emergency room if a careful assessment was not done. Here we see several worrisome signs of impending respiratory failure, including systemic hypertension, tachycardia, increased work of breathing, decrease in cough efficiency, peripheral edema (suggesting possible cor pulmonale), and signs of pulmonary infection (with yellow sputum). If these warning signs were not enough, his admission blood gases with profound hypoxia despite relative alveolar hyperventilation should be of concern. The polycythemia almost certainly reflects chronic hypoxia, and his elevated carboxyhemoglobin level reflects his cigarette smoking.

The *initial assessment* indicates the need for a specific diagnosis of his pulmonary infection (with a sputum culture), conservative treatment of his hypoxemia (with low flow oxygen or Venturi mask), and careful monitoring should intubation and mechanical ventilation be indicated. Before the landmark awareness of oxygen-induced hypoventilation, these patients often ended up on ventilators immediately after their admission to the hospital. Today the use of low flow oxygen therapy and noninvasive mechanical ventilation while bronchial hygiene and antibiotic therapy are at work often makes intubation unnecessary, thus permitting a much less expensive and more comfortable recovery. It is important to note that watchful awareness of both blood pressure and ventilatory status were suggested and certainly indicated.

The *second assessment* occurs in the setting of worsening pulmonary function despite good respiratory care. Clearly the patient has slipped from borderline to overt respiratory failure in the course of his hospitalization. Several points regarding this case are instructive. First, one should note that the patient's complaints became increasingly nonspecific as his blood gases worsened. Indeed in the final assessment the patient's complaints of "feeling worse again" are so nonspecific as to be unhelpful. These nonspecific complaints combined with his increasing lethargy suggest acute respiratory failure.

The blood gases in the *third assessment* confirm ventilatory failure. At that time the patient's pH was 7.28, and his Pa_{CO_2} was 105 mm Hg. The reader should sense that the patient's cough and subjective complaint of dyspnea in the first assessment is helpful to making a diagnosis and should learn that the nonspecific complaints of "I'm having a bad period" and "I'm feeling worse again" really do not help in reaching an accurate assessment as to the nature of the patient's problem.

The next thing to note in this case is the installation by the treating therapist of a series of "watchers" that allow him to monitor the patient closely. At first these consist of his own and the nursing staff's observation, the use of a pulse oximeter, and frequent blood gas analyses. When the patient deteriorates in the last case scenario, he is transferred to the ICU, where again more minute-to-minute observation is possible. At this juncture therapists would do well to ask themselves the following question: What have I done to ensure that this patient is observed carefully in the course of my interface with him?

There are two points in the admitting history worthy of note. One is, as it turns out, a red herring; the other is not. The red herring is the patient's complaint of mild nausea without abdominal pain or vomiting. The therapist notes that the abdominal examination is negative and goes on to other things. Nausea or anorexia complicating chronic obstructive pulmonary disease (COPD) is so common as to be seen in approximately one third of admitted patients. The causes of the nausea can be peptic ulcer disease, aminophylline toxicity, medication effect, or hypoxic bowel syndrome. This patient was not receiving aminophylline-like drugs as an out-patient and was not taking oral steroids. The therapist rightly assesses that the patient does not have significant gastrointestinal obstruction and goes on with his respiratory management of the patient. If he was vomiting or had gastric distension, passing a nasogastric tube would have been helpful.

The fact that the patient had a recent history of depression, persistence in cigarette smoking, and disinterest in pulmonary rehabilitation is missed by the treating therapist here. He fails to ascertain whether the patient has a living will or durable medical power of attorney, information he may wish he had pursued when the patient comes to intubation and commitment to ventilator support.

Note that throughout this case the therapist is appropriately adjusting the patient's oxygen therapy and bronchial hygiene regimen and presumably is using mucolytics. It is not the purpose of this book to specify precisely what treatments need to be ordered. One would imagine, however, that bronchial hygiene or mucolytic therapy every 2 hours by up-draft medication nebulizer might have been used at the start and that this might have been increased to every hour just before the patient's transfer to the ICU. Similarly and appropriately the therapist's initial suggestion of an oxygen Venturi mask to prevent the patient's CO_2 retention from worsening would have been appropriate. Frequent blood gas analyses are requested. The therapist notes that no acute infiltrates are noted on the chest x-ray film and suspects that the patient's hypoxemia may be chronic given his elevated hematocrit. He correctly obtains a sputum sample for culture and contacts the attending physician regarding the need for possible intubation.

Discussion with the physician in this case revealed that prior experience with this patient had suggested that vigorous respiratory care was enough to keep him from having to go on the ventilator. The therapist and physician agreed that they would observe the patient for a few more hours before making that decision. As it turned out, the patient continued to deteriorate and slipped into frank respiratory failure, ultimately requiring intubation.

The consulting therapist's role here is critical in that the monitors that he has set must be acute enough and repeated frequently enough to allow him to evaluate the patient on essentially a minute-to-minute basis. In the final scenario it is standard practice to repeat the chest x-ray examination after intubation to check placement of the endotracheal tube, to determine that a pneumothorax or acute pulmonary infiltrate has not developed, and as a baseline film with the lungs well expanded from deep, respirator-delivered breaths.

⊷ KEY POINT ANSWERS   *For Chronic Bronchitis (DRG 88)*

1. Basic Concept Formation
  a. *Cigarette smoking* and, to a much lesser extent, upper airway infections such as chronic sinusitis, viral infections, and dust and fume exposure.
  b. *Yes.* They are the basis for the approved *definition* of the disease: cough productive of sputum for at least 3 months in 2 consecutive years. These symptoms reflect *stimulation of irritant receptors* in the lung by mucus produced by hypersecreting goblet cells and submucous glands.
  c. Normally by a functioning *mucociliary escalator.* Rarely by *cough.*
  d. *Yes.*
  e. *Absolutely, yes.* Although it may take several months for the total beneficial effect to be appreciated by the patient. (NOTE: The importance of the respiratory care practitioner's role in smoking cessation and other lung health programs cannot be overemphasized.)

2. Data Base Formation
  a. *Mucus hypersecretion, bronchial obstruction,* and some distal air trapping.*
  b. *Airway obstruction producing relative or absolute shunt physiology* (see Fig. 1-8). In addition, stimulation of oxygen receptors, the irritant (cough) reflex, and alveolar hyperinflation account for some of the clinical manifestations.
  c. The *lumen* (secretions) and *wall* (infection and inflammation) (see Fig. 1-3).
  d. *Cyanosis, digital clubbing, erythrocytosis, and cor pulmonale with peripheral edema.*
  e. *Goals:* Reduce inflammation, reduce viscosity of sputum, effect expectoration of mucus, and treat hypoxemia and CO_2 retention. Relieve bronchospasm if present.
  f. *Treatment (TDP selection)*
    (1) *Bronchial Hygiene Therapy Protocol* (see box, p. 6, and Fig. 1-8). For lumen obstruction (see Fig. 1-3): Deep breathing and coughing, suction, mucolytics, airway (aerosol) and systemic hydration, bronchoscopy.
    (2) *Bronchodilator Therapy Protocol* (see box, p. 7, and Fig. 1-7). When wall abnormalities are present (see Fig. 1-3): Systemic antibiotics (physician ordered), antiinflammatory agents, decongestants (rarely).
    (3) *Pulmonary Rehabilitation Protocol* (see Fig. 1-9). For supporting structures: Pursed-lip breathing exercises.
    (4) *Oxygen Therapy Protocol* (see box, p. 6) as needed for hypoxemia.
  g. Protocols' expected outcomes, adverse effects, and monitors:

Protocol	Expected Outcomes	Possible Adverse Effects	Monitors
Bronchial Hygiene (see box, p. 6)	Increased sputum clearance, decreased wheezing	Rare. Percussion and PD may not be tolerated.	Auscultation, sputum findings.
Oxygen Therapy (see box, p. 6)	Improved hypoxemia	CO_2 retention	Spo_2 ABGs

3. Assessment
  a. *Yes.* Dyspnea, productive cough, obstructive physiology on pulmonary function tests (PFTs), physical signs of air trapping, rhonchi, clubbing, hypoxemia, CO_2 retention, and polycythemia.
  b. *Yes.* His ABGs suggested shunt physiology. His polycythemia and edema reflect chronic hypoxemia. His PFT data suggest airway obstruction and air trapping. This was confirmed by his chest physical examination.
  c. The *most worrisome manifestations on admission were* pitting leg edema, tachycardia, hypertension, profound hypoxemia, and moderate CO_2 retention.

4. Application
  a. *Oxygen Therapy* **was** indicated because of the profound hypoxemia and signs of cor pulmonale.
  b. *Monitoring* of heart rate and rhythm, electrocardiogram (ECG) morphology, and pulse oximetry **was** indicated because of the hypoxia. Frequent *level of consciousness checks and sputum volume and consistency* checks also appeared indicated.

*See color plate 2 in Des Jardins T, Burton GG. *Clinical manifestations & assessment of respiratory disease,* ed 3, St Louis, 1995, Mosby.

c. *Bronchial Hygiene Therapy* **was** indicated because of the patient's diagnosis (chronic bronchitis), specifically because of his thick, tenacious secretions.

d. *Percussion and PD* **were** indicated (see 4.c above).

e. If smoking cessation instruction and assistance are part of it, *Pulmonary Rehabilitation* **should** be involved in this patient's care. His use of oxygen and metered dose inhaler (MDI) aerosol therapy should be initiated and evaluated by the pulmonary rehabilitation team.

5. **Evaluation**

   a. Expected *outcomes* of therapy are found in answer 2.g.

   b. Suggested patient *monitors* are found in answer 2.g.

   c. *Limits* of suggested therapies

   (1) *Bronchial Hygiene Therapy:* Mucolytic therapy can be given via aerosol every 2 to 3 hours. Suctioning can be done as often as every 2 to 3 minutes. Percussion and PD are usually not tolerated for more than 30 minutes every 4 hours. Therapeutic bronchoscopy may be done each shift if necessary.

   (2) *Oxygen Therapy:* Upper limit of mask therapy F_{IO_2} (to $F_{IO_2} = 1.0$) will be determined by ABG analysis and by worsening of the patient's CO_2 retention.

   d. *Advantages and Disadvantages of Treatment Modalities:* All are relatively inexpensive (except bronchoscopy) and, with the cautions outlined in answer 2.g, relatively safe. The most cost-effective approach here is *smoking cessation* on the part of the patient.

   e. If the patient *improves,* we would first reduce the F_{IO_2}, then reduce the intensity and frequency of bronchial hygiene therapy, for example, from every 2 to 3 hours to every 4 to 6 hours to every shift.

   f. If *little initial improvement* is seen, early consideration of intubation and therapeutic bronchoscopy is indicated.

6. **Boundary Awareness**

   a. At the time of the *second* assessment the following parameters had worsened or not improved: *heart rate, blood pressure, and ABGs.*

   b. Probably after the *second assessment;* certainly at the time of the *third assessment* because of severe respiratory acidemia.

   c. At the time of the *third assessment* in most clinical settings.

   d. Unrelieved *dyspnea, tachypnea, tachycardia, worsening ABGs,* failure to produce sputum despite intensive therapy (at the time of the *third assessment*).

   e. The possible adverse effects of the treatments selected are presented in 2.g.

CHAPTER 3 Emphysema

RESPONSE 1

S: "I'm so short of breath!"

O: Obvious respiratory distress. Vital signs: BP 155/110, HR 95, RR 25, and T 38.3° C (101° F). Malnourished (66 kg [146 lb], 180 cm [6 ft] tall). Using accessory muscles of inspiration, pursed-lip breathing. Increased anteroposterior chest diameter. Depressed hemidiaphragms and generally diminished breath sounds. Expiration prolonged. Crackles in right lower lobe. CXR: apical scarring, large bleb in right middle lobe, pulmonary hyperexpansion, right lower lobe infiltrate consistent with pneumonia. Cough: weak and productive of small amount of yellow sputum. ABGs (on 2 L/min O_2 by nasal cannula): pH 7.59, $Paco_2$ 40, HCO_3^- 37, and Pao_2 38.

A: • Bronchitic exacerbation of COPD (history, general appearance, ABGs, CXR)
  • Increased work of breathing (increased respiratory rate, blood pressure, and heart rate)
  • Alveolar infiltrate in right lower lobe; presumed lobar pneumonia (CXR, fever)
  • Excessive bronchial secretions and poor ability to mobilize them (yellow sputum and weak cough)
  • Acute alveolar hyperventilation superimposed on chronic ventilatory failure with severe hypoxemia (ABGs and history)
    • Impending ventilatory failure
  • Presumed malnutrition

P: Oxygen therapy per protocol (careful not to knock out hypoxic drive to breath). Bronchial hygiene therapy per protocol (including a sputum culture). Trial of bronchodilator therapy per protocol. Have mechanical ventilator on standby. Monitor closely (e.g., every hour, vital signs, pulse oximetry, ABGs). When patient is ready to be discharged, schedule a patient and family education session—including nutrition consult.

RESPONSE 2

S: "My chest feels tighter, and I'm more short of breath."

O: Vital signs: BP 160/115, HR 97, RR 15 and shallow, T = 37.8° C (100° F). May be getting fatigued (e.g., no use of accessory muscles of inspiration); diminished breath sounds; no air entry may be the reason for no crackles in right lower lobe. ABGs: pH 7.28, $Paco_2$ 82, HCO_3^- 36, and Pao_2 41. Pulse oximetry: 68%.

A: • Continued increase in respiratory distress and fatigue (blood pressure, heart rate, shallow respiratory rate, no use of accessory muscles)
  • Right lower lobe infiltrate (dull percussion notes and admission CXR).
  • Acute ventilatory failure superimposed on chronic ventilatory failure with severe hypoxemia ($Paco_2$ higher and pH lower than patient's normal baseline; general patient fatigue)

P: Call physician stat regarding acute ventilatory failure; recommend transfer to ICU and mechanical ventilation per protocol (adjust tidal volume and ventilatory rate until the patient's normal $Paco_2$ and pH are achieved). Up-regulate oxygen therapy per ventilator protocol. Up-regulate bronchial hygiene therapy per protocol. Continue trial period of bronchodilator therapy per protocol. Monitor closely and reevaluate after patient is intubated and placed on ventilator.

Discussion

The student will recall that emphysema is a slowly progressive *destructive* process involving lung parenchyma. In the case of panacinar (panlobular) emphysema the loss of pulmonary function may be as much as 60 to 100 cc of FEV_1 per year. More rapid declines in pulmonary function are accompanied by conditions known to exacerbate COPD (e.g., acute bronchitis, pneumonia, pneumothorax). In this case the patient's fever, history of a flulike syndrome, crackles in the right lower lobe, and a right lower lobe infiltrate on x-ray film all point to an acute pneumonia as reason for his deterioration. It should be stressed that a correct response in this case was the rapid obtaining of a Gram stain and culture of the sputum.

A "red herring" in this case is the patient's earlier reported failure to improve with bronchodilator therapy. Any exacerbation of COPD deserves an in-hospital trial of aggressive bronchial hygiene and bronchodilator therapy, since reversible bronchospasm may be one of the only components of the deterioration that will respond. Accordingly, putting the patient on an up-draft nebulizer treatment with bronchodilator, encouraging deep breathing and coughing, and use of mucolytics and systemic hydration are all indicated in this case, even though they had been of little use in the past.

It is a good call for the treating team to recognize the patient's malnutrition, to quantitatively assess it, and to bring early professional attention to the condition while he is in the hospital for this pneumonic exacerbation.

The fact that the patient would suddenly (at the time of the *second assessment*) slip into acute respiratory failure with significant CO_2 retention is not surprising. In some series of such patients this occurs more than 50% of the time, despite judicious use of oxygen and entirely appropriate respiratory care otherwise.

It should be noted that the patient had previously requested that "no heroics" be used on him, but the attending physician was able to convince the patient to accept a period of mechanical ventilation when his clinical condition deteriorated despite the initial aggressive therapy prescribed. The organism responsible for this exacerbation (pneumococcus) was subsequently identified, and the patient gradually improved as antibiotic therapy and ventilator support were continued for a 10-day hospital stay. The patient was discharged on dietary supplementation and a program of multiple small feedings.

Attention must be drawn to the fact of the decreased adventitious breath sounds in the right lower lobe at the second assessment. The reader who correctly assumed that this was due to decreased air entry in an airless, possibly obstructed right lower lobe should be congratulated. The fact that the crackles go away within 6 hours of admission does *not* suggest that the patient is improving. Indeed it suggests just the opposite, as evidenced by the patient's deteriorating arterial blood gas values!

CHAPTER 4 Bronchiectasis

S: Complaints of constant dyspnea and productive cough.

O: Cyanotic, mild digital clubbing. Pursed-lip breathing and using accessory muscles of inspiration. Frequent, strong cough. Large amounts of foul smelling, yellow-green sputum. Vital signs: BP 185/90, HR 110, RR 30, T 37.9° C (100.2° F). Bilateral rhonchi and crackles. PFT: mild-to-moderate degree of airway obstruction. Bedside PEFR: 325. ABGs (on 3 L/min O_2 nc): pH 7.52, Pa_{CO_2} 35, HCO_3^- 27, Pa_{O_2} 53. CXR: cystic bronchiectasis, moderate alveolar hyperinflation, increased markings.

A: • Respiratory distress (general appearance, vital signs, pursed-lip breathing, use of accessory muscles)
• Excessive bronchial secretions (cough, sputum, rhonchi, and crackles)
 • Infection likely (yellow-green sputum)
• Acute alveolar hyperventilation superimposed on chronic ventilatory failure with mild hypoxemia (ABGs)
 • Possible impending ventilatory failure

P: Bronchial hygiene therapy per protocol (obtain sputum culture). Oxygen therapy per protocol. Monitor possible impending ventilatory failure closely (e.g., vital signs, ABGs, pulse oximeter). Reevaluate frequently.

S: "I've been short of breath for several hours."

O: Cyanotic, pursed-lip breathing and using accessory muscles of respiration. Frequent cough, producing large amounts of foul smelling, bloody, yellow-green secretions. Sputum culture: *Streptococcus* and *P. aeruginosa*. Vital signs: BP 188/95, HR 118, RR 34, T normal. Bilateral rhonchi and crackles. Bronchial breath sounds over the RLL. Sp_{O_2}: 93%. ABGs: pH 7.54, Pa_{CO_2} 30, HCO_3^- 28, Pa_{O_2} 57. CXR: RLL atelectasis or pneumonic infiltrate.

A: • Continued respiratory distress (general appearance, vital signs, pursed-lip breathing, use of accessory muscles)
• Excessive bronchial secretions (cough, sputum, rhonchi and crackles)
• Right lower lobe atelectasis vs. pneumonia/consolidation (CXR, bronchial breath sounds)
• Acute alveolar hyperventilation superimposed on chronic ventilatory failure with mild hypoxemia (ABGs)
 • Possible impending ventilatory failure

P: Up-regulate bronchial hygiene therapy per protocol. Up-regulate oxygen therapy per protocol. Start hyperinflation therapy per protocol. Continue to monitor impending ventilatory failure. Reevaluate.

RESPONSE 3

S: "I'm breathing much better."

O: Strong cough. Sputum: moderate amount of thin, clear secretions. Vital signs: BP 135/80, HR 80, RR 14, T normal. Mild-to-moderate rhonchi and crackles over both lung bases. Spo_2: 94%. ABGs: pH 7.48, $Paco_2$ 49, HCO_3^- 38, Pao_2 66. CXR: opacity no longer present in RLL. No other acute infiltrates.

A:
- Respiratory distress no longer present (patient's comment, vital signs, ABGs)
- Bronchial secretions (thin, clear secretions)
  - Infection appears to be improving
- Atelectasis/pneumonia improving (CXR, ABGs)
- Acute alveolar hyperventilation on top of chronic ventilatory failure with mild hypoxemia: improving (ABGs)
  - Impending ventilatory failure no longer present

P: Down-regulate bronchial hygiene therapy per protocol. Continue oxygenation therapy per protocol. Discontinue hyperinflation therapy per protocol. Monitor and reevaluate.

Discussion

Although increasingly rare in clinical practice, bronchiectasis is one of the chronic lung diseases with which the respiratory care practitioner must be familiar. It presents as recurrent pulmonary infections with variable pulmonary scarring over the years. The pathophysiology is similar to that of cystic fibrosis in that frequently secretions are retained and there is right-to-left intrapulmonary shunting.

This patient was already known to the medical center as having bronchiectasis, and this certainly made her care more straightforward. The bilateral rhonchi and crackles heard on the *first assessment* clearly suggest a need for the bronchial hygiene therapy that was performed. This therapy must include postural drainage and percussion therapy as well as mucolysis. As in all obstructive pulmonary diseases, a trial of bronchodilator therapy in-hospital certainly would not be out of order. The sputum often produces organisms such as seen here (*Streptococcus* and *Pseudomonas*), and a sputum culture is appropriate.

Of most concern was the patient's initial blood gas values, which had deteriorated from those 2 years earlier. Most significantly, her drop in Pao_2 from 68 mm Hg on 2 L/min O_2 to 53 mm Hg on 3 L/min was worrisome. Note that no frank pneumonic infiltrate was noted on the initial chest x-ray film but that one did appear in the right lower lobe on the third hospital day. This infiltrate could have been from atelectasis due to proximal airway mucus plugging or, alternatively, from an acute pneumonia. The treatments for these conditions are not all that different in that the airway obstruction must be relieved and the appropriate antibiotics given.

Note that on the *second assessment* the patient is seen to be developing severe hypoxemia despite any oxygen therapy the therapist would have selected. A trial of 50% oxygen via a Venturi mask is indicated. One can argue that hyperinflation therapy was not indicated here. If the right lower lobe infiltrate was atelectatic, such therapy would certainly be indicated, and we have no quarrel with it on a trial basis in this case, after the second assessment.

The *last assessment* shows that vigorous therapy pays off. The patient appears to be improving nicely, and the infiltrate in the right lower lobe has disappeared. This strongly suggests that the cause of the infiltrate was postobstructive atelectasis and not pneumonia.

What was *not* included in the final assessment and plan was an injunction to assess the patient's knowledge of her respiratory hygiene program. Specifically, this should include a review of her knowledge of the first signs of pulmonary infection and of the methodology for any aerosol devices that had been described. Certainly a review and instructions for herself and her caregivers in chest percussion and postural drainage techniques is in order.

CHAPTER 5   Asthma

RESPONSE 1

S: "I feel horrible, and my chest feels tight."

O: Pursed-lip breathing. Cyanotic. Using accessory muscles of inspiration. Frequent, strong cough productive of moderate amount of thick, white mucus. Vital signs: BP 110/85, HR 190, RR 28, afebrile. Bilateral diminished breath sounds, wheezing, and rhonchi. PEFR: 150. CXR: air trapping and depressed diaphragm. Spo_2 (2 L/min O_2 by cannula): 77%. ABGs: pH 7.45, $Paco_2$ 28, HCO_3^- 19, Pao_2 40.

A: • Status asthmaticus (general history and clinical data)
 • Increased work of breathing (HR, RR, and use of accessory muscles).
 • Bronchospasm (wheezing and PEFR)
 • Excessive bronchial secretions but effective cough (sputum production)
 • Acute alveolar hyperventilation and metabolic acidosis with severe hypoxemia (lactic acid causing pH and HCO_3^- to be lower than expected for an acute decrease in $Paco_2$ level)
   • Possible impending ventilatory failure

P: Up-regulate oxygen therapy per protocol. Aggressive bronchodilator therapy per protocol. Bronchial hygiene therapy per protocol. Continue beclomethasone inhaler as prescribed for home use. Contact physician regarding impending ventilatory failure. Monitor and reevaluate continuously (e.g., vital signs, breath sounds, pulse oximetry, ABGs, and PEFR every 15 to 30 minutes). Place ventilator on standby and prepare for intubation if patient is not improved.

RESPONSE 2

S: "I'm sorry. I'm wheezing too much, and I can't go to sleep."

O: Pursed-lip breathing. Cyanotic. Using accessory muscles of inspiration. Frequent, strong cough. Moderate amount of thick, white mucus. PEFR: 175. Vital signs: BP 105/82, HR 180, RR 24. Prolonged expiration. Bilateral diminished breath sounds, wheezing, and rhonchi. Spo_2: 95%. ABGs: pH 7.48, $Paco_2$ 34, HCO_3^- 24, Pao_2 73.

A: • Continued increased work of breathing (vital signs, use of accessory muscles, ABGs)
 • Bronchospasm (wheezing and PEFR)
 • Thick bronchial secretions (sputum production)
 • Acute alveolar hyperventilation with mild hypoxemia improving (lactic acidosis corrected)
   • Impending ventilatory failure still possible

P: Continue or up-regulate oxygen therapy per protocol. Continue bronchodilator therapy per protocol. Up-regulate bronchial hygiene therapy per protocol. Continue beclomethasone inhaler as prescribed for home use. Continue to maintain ventilator on standby. Continue to monitor and reevaluate closely.

RESPONSE 3

S: "I feel like there is a weight on my chest."

O: Using accessory muscles. Pursed-lip breathing. Skin: damp, cool, and cyanotic. No cough or sputum. PEFR: 145. Vital signs: BP 160/100, HR 185, RR 13. Diminished breath sounds bilaterally. No wheezing or rhonchi noted. Spo_2: 79%. ABGs: pH 7.27, $Paco_2$ 57, HCO_3^- 24, Pao_2 51.

A: • Patient is becoming fatigued (no wheezing, vital signs, ABGs)
 • Worsening bronchospasm ("silent chest," with decreased wheezing and decreased sputum production)
 • Acute ventilatory failure with moderate hypoxemia (ABGs)

P: Contact physician stat. Consider mechanical ventilation. Up-regulate oxygen therapy per protocol (e.g., using a Venturi mask). Up-regulate bronchodilator therapy per protocol. Up-regulate bronchial hygiene therapy per protocol (aggressive). Continue beclomethasone inhaler as prescribed for home use. Monitor and reevaluate continuously—every 15 to 30 minutes.

Discussion

The historical point that the patient not only has asthma but also has had it severely enough recently to require hospitalizations and ventilator interfaces is important and should alert the respiratory care practitioner to the fact that he is dealing with more than the run-of-the-mill asthmatic. The fact that the patient's mother has stopped smoking, made environmental changes at home, and has been faithful enough to have the child on a home recording program of peak expiratory flow rates and that the child has been desensitized speak to a compliant and intelligent patient and family.

The pursed-lip breathing, cyanosis, prolonged expirations, use of accessory muscles of respiration, frequent cough, thick, white mucus, increased heart rate and blood pressure, and the severity of the child's hypoxemia (despite alveolar hyperventilation on admission) are all good severity indicators and suggest that vigorous therapy will be necessary. Many workers feel that sputum and blood eosinophilia is a good marker for allergic exacerbations of asthma. A circulating eosinophil count or Wright's stain for sputum eosinophilia, or both, might have been in order.

Note in Response 1 that the pH and HCO_3^- levels are lower than expected for a particular Pa_{CO_2} level. This is most likely because of the *lactic acid* caused by the severe hypoxemia. The lactic acid offsets the increased pH and HCO_3^- levels that should develop immediately in response to an acutely decreased Pa_{CO_2} level—according to the P_{CO_2}-HCO_3^--pH nomogram (a Pa_{CO_2} of 28 should move the pH to a level greater than 7.52). The patient's ABGs (pH 7.45, Pa_{CO_2} 28, HCO_3^- 19, and Pa_{O_2} 40) are often *incorrectly* interpretated as *chronic alveolar hyperventilation with hypoxemia.*

In this case the following *two* primary indicators confirm that the patient has acute alveolar hyperventilation with hypoxemia and not chronic alveolar hyperventilation: (1) the patient's age and history of acute asthmatic episodes and (2) the severe hypoxemia. Because of the increased work of breathing (vital signs) and acute alveolar hyperventilation, the possibility of impending ventilatory failure is real.

At this point, however, the child is not retaining CO_2, so increasing the nasal oxygen therapy to 4 L/min or, alternatively, using a Venturi mask is reasonable. The child needs frequent bronchodilator and inhaled steroid therapy, and this should have been started. The semicritical nature of her illness and impending ventilatory failure should have been reported to the physician immediately after the first assessment. Intravenous corticosteroid medications are almost always used in this setting. Increasingly, continuous nebulized bronchodilator therapy is used in children such as this.

At the time of the *second assessment* we are more than 2 hours into aggressive therapy. It appears that the patient is improving slightly. The physical findings have changed little, and there is still mild hypoxemia. Assuming the student correctly increased the patient's oxygen therapy after the first assessment, a key point to note here is that hypoxemia is present despite oxygen therapy. It would be safe to further increase the oxygen therapy. Use of a nonrebreathing oxygen mask would be appropriate. Hydration of the patient (and her secretions) would be helpful, probably via the parenteral route. Close monitoring of vital signs, pulse oximetry, breath sounds, and PEFR and judicious use of arterial or capillary sample blood gas analyses should continue.

By the time of the *final case scenario* (Response 3), it is clear that the patient's status asthmaticus has worsened to the point of acute ventilatory failure. There is now significant CO_2 retention and persistent severe hypoxemia. The silent chest does not represent improved bronchoconstriction. Rather, it suggests that there has been a marked diminution of gas flow, so that breath sounds are no longer generated. Confirmation in this regard comes from the fact that the patient can no longer cough up secretions. Presumably they too are being expectorated with difficulty, given the obstructed airway. A chest x-ray film to rule out bilateral pneumothorax as a cause of the bilaterally diminished breath sounds is a good idea.

The therapist at this point should not leave the patient and should be prepared to bag and mask or (if it is allowed in the individual institution) to go ahead with emergency intubation. The patient's hypertension and tachycardia suggest that further administration of bronchodilator aerosol alone is contraindicated, unless or until the patient has a mechanically open airway.

➔ KEY POINT ANSWERS | *For Asthma (DRG 98)*

1. Basic Concept Formation

a. *Yes.* True bronchial asthma, triggered by exposure to *extrinsic antigens,* commonly begins in childhood. It frequently is associated with other symptoms of allergy, such as *allergic rhinitis* (hay fever) or hives.

b. *Yes.* Although less commonly than children. In adults the asthma is often *not* related to extrinsic allergy such as pollen, dust, and danders. Often it follows bouts of respiratory infection. It is called *intrinsic asthma,* or asthmatic bronchitis.

c. *Yes.* The main pathophysiologic mechanisms activated in asthma are *airway inflammation and hyperreactivity,* resulting in mucus *hypersecretion and bronchoconstriction.*

d. *Not necessarily.* The patient or his caregiver is required to *assess and treat* his condition, much as the respiratory care practitioner practicing in the therapist-driven protocol (TDP) paradigm. Multiple therapeutic strategies and modalities are often required to achieve good "control" of the patient's symptoms. Even with optimal outpatient and home care, exacerbations of asthma may require patient visits to the emergency department or hospitalization.

e. *No. Dyspnea and wheezing* are the most common symptoms of asthma.

f. *Yes.* See 1.d (above). Such analysis and treatment selection by the patient or his caregiver are the basis for the NAEP (National Asthma Education Project) Guidelines.*

g. Inhaled *antiallergic or antiinflammatory agents* such as cromolyn sodium, nedocromil, or inhaled steroids and beta-agonist and anticholinergic bronchodilator aerosols. Avoidance of allergens and immunotherapy (desensitization injections) are other avenues of approach.

h. As with pneumothorax, massive pulmonary embolism, and foreign body aspiration, asthma often presents fairly acutely with a *crisis onset* over a few minutes or hours. Symptoms may abate as quickly as they arose. About 50% of asthmatic children seem to outgrow their asthma by the time of puberty. By adulthood, more than 75% of childhood asthmatics are greatly improved or no longer symptomatic.

2. Data Base Formation

a. Asthma is a chronic lung disease characterized by airway obstruction and narrowing (which may or may not be reversible), airway inflammation, and airway hyperresponsiveness to a variety of stimuli. Airway smooth muscle contraction and mucus hypersecretion that causes airway obstruction are the primary abnormalities in asthma.†

b. The commonly recognized *types* of asthma are classified by their triggers:
   (1) Extrinsic asthma. See 1.b (above).
   (2) Intrinsic asthma (asthmatic bronchitis). See 1.b (above).
   (3) Exercise-induced asthma.
   (4) Cough-variant asthma.
   (5) Cold-induced asthma.
   (6) Fume- or vapor-induced asthma (reactive airway disease).
   (7) Catamenial (menses-related) asthma.

c. *Increased airway resistance and decreased $\dot{V}/\dot{Q}$ (shunt)* are the primary pathophysiologic mechanisms responsible for the *clinical manifestations* of asthma (see Fig. 1-7). *Air trapping, retained or excessive secretions,* and *chemoreceptor discharge* are secondary mechanisms involved.

d. The airway model (see Fig. 1-3) consists of airway wall, lumen, and supporting structures. The wall and lumen components are abnormal in asthma. Some investigators believe that the supporting structures, that is, the lung parenchyma, may also be abnormal in chronic asthma.

e. According to the NAEP Guidelines, effective management of asthma, which can prevent exacerbations, relies on *four essential components,* each with separate goals:
   (1) Objective measures of lung function to *assess and monitor* the *severity* of the asthma exacerbation.

---

*NAEP: Guidelines for the diagnosis and management of asthma. DHHS Expert Panel Report, 1991.
†See color plate 6 in Des Jardins T, Burton GG: *Clinical manifestations & assessment of respiratory disease,* ed 3, St. Louis, 1995, Mosby.

(2) Pharmacologic therapy to *relieve symptoms* by reducing airway inflammation.

(3) Environmental measures to *control allergens and irritants*.

(4) Patient education to *improve patient knowledge of his disease*.

Patient education should include efforts to educate the patient's family. Parent, teacher, and community education is important for the proper diagnosis and management of asthma in pediatric and adolescent patients. *Good control* of asthma results in shorter, less frequent, and less severe exacerbations, fewer trips to the doctor's office or hospital, and longer symptom-free intervals between asthmatic attacks.

f. *Treatment* (TDP selection)

(1) *Bronchial Hygiene Therapy Protocol* (see Fig. 1-8 and box, p. 6). For lumen obstruction, see airway model, Fig. 1-3: Deep breathing and coughing, suctioning, airway (bland aerosol) and systemic hydration, and occasionally therapeutic bronchoscopy.

(2) *Bronchodilator Therapy Protocol* (see Fig. 1-7 and box, p. 7) For wall abnormalities, see airway model, Fig. 1-3: Aerosolized *antiinflammatory* agents (corticosteroids and nonsteroidal antiinflammatory agents such as cromolyn and nedocromil) and, rarely, decongestants.

(3) *Oxygen Therapy Protocol* (see box, p. 6) as needed for hypoxemia.

g. Modalities' typical therapies ordered, expected outcomes, and monitors:

Modality	Typical Therapies Ordered	Expected Outcomes	Monitors
Oxygen therapy (see box, p. 6)	Oxygen per nasal cannula 4 L/min	Increased Pao_2, Spo_2; normalizing $Paco_2$, heart rate, respiratory rate	$Spo_2 \geq 92\%$; ECG
Bronchodilator therapy (see box, p. 7)	Proventil, 0.2 ml in 2 ml normal saline q30min × 3	Less dyspnea, less wheezing, improved ease of expectoration	$Spo_2 \geq 92\%$; improved PEFR
Antiinflammatory aerosol therapy	Beclovent 4 puffs q2h × 4	See modality above	See modality above
Bronchial hygiene therapy (see box, p. 6)	Postural drainage, chest physical therapy, cough and deep breathe q4h	See bronchodilator therapy above	See bronchodilator therapy above; increased sputum production

3. Assessment

a. *Yes.* The symptoms of an acute asthma exacerbation included episodic, worsening *dyspnea* and (to a lesser extent) *cough* productive of thick, tenacious sputum. The signs of asthma, that is its *clinical manifestations,* include her falling PEFR, her appearance ("tripod" stance, pursed-lip breathing, barrel chest deformity, use of accessory muscles, and cyanosis), rapid heart and respiratory rate, findings on chest auscultation (wheezes and rhonchi), and laboratory findings (hyperinflation on chest x-ray, hypoxemia in ABGs, and obstructive physiology demonstration on PFTs).

b. *Yes.* The initial signs and symptoms in this case, especially when taken with the history, are practically pathognomonic of the pathophysiologic mechanisms seen in asthma (see Fig. 1-7). Signs are as follows:

(1) Falling PEFR; wheezes suggest *increased airway resistance.*

(2) Appearance (tripod stance, pursed-lip breathing, barrel chest, use of accessory muscles) suggests *increased work of breathing.*

(3) Cyanosis and hypoxemia on ABGs reflect *shunt physiology.*

(4) Rapid heart rate, labored, rapid breathing, and chest tightness suggest *cardiopulmonary distress* and *hypoxemia.*

(5) Diminished breath sounds, wheezing, rhonchi, and air trapping on her admission chest x-ray film suggest *increased airway resistance and alveolar hyperinflation.*

c. The *initial indications of severity* in this case include impending ventilatory failure, severe breathlessness, cough, chest tightness, wheezing in a relatively silent chest, tachycardia, tachypnea, use of accessory muscles, cyanosis, and profound hypoxemia on supplemental oxygen despite alveolar hyperventilation.

4. Application

a. Oxygen therapy **was** indicated because of the patient's severe hypoxemia.

b. Monitoring of heart rate, rhythm, ECG morphology, ABGs and pulse oximetry **was** indicated because of the patient's severe respiratory distress, tachycardia, and hypoxemia.

  c. Bronchial hygiene therapy **was** indicated because of the need for mucolysis and expectoration to clear mucus in her obstructed airways. Postural drainage and chest percussion *may have been tried* to aid in expectoration of thick, tenacious secretions. This modality is often not tolerated during severe asthmatic exacerbations.

  d. Bronchodilator and antiinflammatory aerosol therapy **were** indicated because of her diagnosis of *bronchial asthma* with wheezing.

  e. Hyperinflation therapy **was not** indicated because the patient had no evidence of atelectasis and already demonstrated air trapping.

  f. Intubation and mechanical ventilation **were not** indicated, as the other therapies (see a to d above) had not yet been tried, and the patient was under close observation.

5. Evaluation

  a. Expected *outcomes* of therapy are listed in answer 2.g.

  b. Suggested parameters to *monitor* are listed in 2.g.

  c. Limits of suggested therapies:

   (1) *Bronchial Hygiene Therapy:* Bland aerosol therapy is not tolerated at all by many asthmatics, and mucolytics such as acetylcysteine are relatively contraindicated because of their tendency to cause or worsen airway inflammation and to cause bronchospasm. Suctioning may be done as frequently as tolerated (as much as every 2 to 3 minutes) and percussion and PD are generally not tolerated well at all. Therapeutic bronchoscopy may be done as frequently as new, otherwise untreatable atelectasis develops distal to obstructive airways.

   (2) *Bronchodilator Therapy:* May be given (under close monitoring of heart rate) *continuously* in status asthmaticus. Anti-inflammatory therapy may initially be given via aerosol every hour, then every 3 to 4 hours.

   (3) *Oxygen Therapy:* The upper limit of nasal cannula oxygen therapy is 5 to 6 L/min; mask F_{IO_2} may be increased to 1.0 as determined by repeat ABG analysis and is limited by CO_2 retention.

  d. *Advantages of Treatment Modalities:* All are relatively inexpensive (except bronchoscopy) and, with the monitors outlined in 2.g (above), relatively safe. The most cost-effective approach over the long term is *prevention of exacerbations,* which appears to have been attempted in this patient right along. If because of the patient's metabolic acidosis the reader has elected *initially* to intubate and *mechanically ventilate* the patient, the benefits and adverse effects of that modality (e.g., barotrauma) should be reviewed.

  e. If the patient *improves,* first reduce the F_{IO_2} and frequency of aerosolized bronchodilator treatments. Wait 24 to 48 hours before greatly reducing the frequency of administration of her aerosolized steroids to less than every 4 to 6 hours.

  f. If *little improvement* occurs with oxygen, bronchial hygiene, and bronchodilator and antiinflammatory aerosol therapy, we would not hesitate to quickly intubate and mechanically ventilate this patient. If atelectasis were present, we would probably bronchoscope and intubate her at the same time.

6. Boundary Awareness

  a. At the time of the *second* assessment the following parameters had worsened or not significantly improved: heart rate and apparent *persistent increased work of breathing.* Her ABGs looked better, although to know this for sure, it is necessary to calculate the A-a oxygen gradient.

  b. *Yes.* The patient can be shown how to assess her own symptoms and peak flow rates. The caregiver can be instructed in assessment of the severity of her daughter's symptoms and in the use of new modalities if applicable.

  c. Probably a supervisor should have been asked for help at the time of the *first* assessment. Children with status asthmaticus are virtually never "no code," and aggressive care will, generally, be required by all concerned. This child is acutely ill, in impending ventilatory failure, and probably will be transferred to an ICU. Certainly a supervisor should have been consulted by the time of the *third* assessment, when acute ventilatory failure has occurred.

  d. Depending on the physician's preference in such cases, certainly he or she should have been called by the time of the *third* assessment. In fact, many respiratory care protocols state that the physician should be notified when ventilatory failure is impending.

  e. *Ventilatory failure* is diagnosed on the basis of resistant hypoxemia and progressive CO_2 retention with acidemia.

f. Severe asthma, which is episodic by definition, may progress to continuous asthma, which is called *status asthmaticus.* Unless this is terminated quickly, ventilatory failure will develop. Spontaneous pneumothorax may complicate asthma, or it may be a result of ventilator-induced *barotrauma.* Hypercorticism secondary to corticosteroid therapy may also occur, although not usually as a result of *aerosolized* steroid therapy. *Tachycardia* and *cardiac arrhythmias* may result from excessive beta-stimulant bronchodilator therapy.

CHAPTER 6   Cystic Fibrosis

RESPONSE 1

S: "I've not been this short of breath in a long time."

O: Skin: pale and cyanotic. Barrel chest and using accessory muscles of respiration. Digital clubbing. Cough frequent and productive. Sputum: sweet smelling, thick, yellow-green. Distended neck veins and peripheral edema. Vital signs: RR 28, BP 142/90, HR 108, T normal. Bilateral hyperresonant percussion notes. Diminished breath sounds. Crackles and rhonchi. CXR: hyperlucency, flattened diaphragm, and right ventricular enlargement. ABGs (1.5 L/min O_2 by nc): pH 7.51, $Paco_2$ 58, HCO_3^- 43, Pao_2 66. Spo_2 94%.

A: • Respiratory distress (general appearance, vital signs)
   • Excessive tracheobronchial tree secretions (productive cough)
     • Infection likely (yellow-green sputum)
   • Hyperinflated alveoli (barrel chest, use of accessory muscles, CXR)
   • Acute alveolar hyperventilation superimposed on chronic ventilatory failure with mild hypoxemia (history, ABGs)
     • Possible impending ventilatory failure
   • Cor pulmonale (distended neck veins, peripheral edema, CXR)

P: Bronchial hygiene therapy per protocol (including a sputum culture). Oxygenation therapy per protocol. Monitor possible impending ventilatory failure closely (e.g., pulse oximetry, vital signs, ABGs).

RESPONSE 2

S: "I can't get enough air to sleep 10 minutes!"

O: Cyanotic and using accessory muscles of respiration. Vital signs: RR 32, BP 147/95, HR 117, T normal. Cough: frequent, weak, and productive of large amounts of thick, green sputum. *Pseudomonas aeruginosa* cultured. Bilateral hyperresonant notes and diminished breath sounds; crackles, rhonchi, and wheezes. Spo_2: 92%. ABGs: pH 7.55, $Paco_2$ 54, HCO_3^- 45, Pao_2 57.

A: • Continued respiratory distress (general appearance, vital signs, use of accessory muscles)
   • Excessive bronchial secretions (cough, sputum, breath sounds)
     • Poor ability to mobilize secretions (weak cough)
   • Acute alveolar hyperventilation superimposed on chronic ventilatory failure with mild-to-moderate hypoxemia, (ABGs)
     • Possible impending ventilatory failure

P: Up-regulate bronchial hygiene therapy per protocol. Up-regulate oxygenation therapy per protocol. Continue to monitor possible impending ventilatory failure closely.

RESPONSE 3

S: "I can't get into a comfortable position to breathe."

O: Cyanotic. Pursed-lip breathing and using accessory muscles of respiration. Vital signs: RR 22, BP 145/90, HR 120. Bilateral hyperresonant percussion notes, crackles, rhonchi, and wheezing. Spo_2: 65%. ABGs: pH 7.33, $Paco_2$ 79, HCO_3^- 41, Pao_2 37.

A: • Continued respiratory distress (general appearance, vital signs, use of accessory muscles, pursed-lip breathing)
   • Excessive bronchial secretions (cough, sputum, breath sounds)

- Acute ventilatory failure superimposed on chronic ventilatory failure with severe hypoxemia. (ABGs, vital signs)

P: Contact physician stat. Consider mechanical ventilation. Up-regulate bronchial hygiene therapy per protocol. Up-regulate oxygenation therapy per protocol. Monitor closely.

Discussion

The science of respiratory care has advanced over the years, and the prognosis for patients with this multisystem genetic disorder has improved. In our own lifetime at least four therapeutic landmarks can be noted:

1. Vigorous use of chest physical therapy (percussion and postural drainage)
2. Intermittent treatment of secretions with antibiotics and mucolytic enzymes, such as rhDNase
3. Positive expiratory pressure (PEP) therapy
4. Lung transplantation (when all else fails)

This patient had received at least two of these treatments and was in the hands of caring parents. His own indomitable nature and interest in athletics was clearly helpful in his prolonged survival. It is important to note the circumstances surrounding his *admission,* especially that he had experienced hemoptysis, dyspnea, and weight loss during the period preceding his admission. Note also that he had started smoking cigarettes.

In this case we have purposely buried his chief complaints in the admitting history. The reader should have discerned from it that the patient was coughing productively, had hemoptysis, dyspnea, and weight loss. Our recommended therapeutic strategy arises out of recognition of these four presenting complaints. Note also that on admission the patient presented with neck vein distension and peripheral edema, suggesting cor pulmonale. If the experience with chronic obstructive pulmonary disease can be translated to patients with cystic fibrosis, this is a bad prognostic sign and one that clearly calls for intensification of the therapeutic regimen.

Note that on the initial physical examination there were no baseline arterial blood gases with which to compare. Thus the observation of an elevated $Paco_2$ should be taken very, very seriously, since it is not clear (at least initially) whether this is a "chronic" arterial blood gas value or not.

At the time of the *second evaluation* the patient is clearly not improving. Bronchial hygiene therapy now might consist of increasing chest physical therapy to every hour as tolerated, increasing bronchodilator and mucolytic therapy to every 2 hours, and even considering bronchoscopy. If it had not been done earlier, monitoring of ECG and pulse oximetry must be done now. A repeat chest x-ray film would not be out of order at this time. At this point, consider that the patient may have an element of metabolic alkalosis, secondary to his malnutrition, diuretic use, or previous nausea and vomiting. The pH is high and is interfering with release of his already low arterial oxygen to tissues.

The *third assessment* suggests that the patient is clearly deteriorating despite vigorous noninvasive therapy. At this point the patient might be put on a high-concentration Venturi mask, but he probably should be intubated and ventilated. The addition of mechanical ventilation at this time prevents fatigue, allows deep nasal tracheal suctioning, and if necessary facilitates repeat bronchoscopy.

Despite this initial downhill course the patient did improve and was finally extubated. It is hoped the therapist will remember that despite all the "good" things the patient and family had done to treat his illness, the initiation of the smoking habit (on the part of the patient) clearly could be a "last straw" phenomenon. The patient should be placed on a smoking cessation program. This step is as important for the long-term prognosis as is the skill of the practitioner caring for him during this bout of acute ventilatory failure.

CHAPTER **7** Croup Syndrome

RESPONSE 1

S: None available (patient crying).

O: Respiratory distress: inspiratory stridor, brassy cough, HR 160, BP 110/70, RR 58, T normal, intercostal and supraclavicular retractions. Diminished breath sounds. Spo_2 (O_2 mask): 88%.

A: • Croup (moderate to severe) (history, inspiratory stridor)

P: Oxygen therapy per protocol. Cool mist aerosol treatment and mist tent per protocol. Aerosolized racemic epinephrine per protocol. Throat culture. Monitor closely.

RESPONSE 2

S: Wants to go home.

O: Respiratory distress: inspiratory stridor, brassy cough, HR 155, BP 146/88, RR 63, intercostal and supraclavicular retractions. Diminished breath sounds. Spo_2: 90%. Lateral neck x-ray film: subglottic haziness.

A: • Croup (moderate to severe) (history, inspiratory stridor, neck x-ray film)
• Persistent hypoxemia (Spo_2)

P: Up-regulate oxygen therapy per protocol. Up-regulate cool mist aerosol treatment and mist tent per protocol. Up-regulate aerosolized racemic epinephrine per protocol. Monitor closely.

RESPONSE 3

S: Nods that he feels better.

O: Inspiratory stridor and supraclavicular retractions are no longer present. Vital signs. BP 125/80, HR 89, RR 15. Normal breath sounds. Spo_2: 97%.

A: • Subglottic edema no longer present

P: Reduce or discontinue oxygen therapy per protocol. Discontinue the aerosol cool mist treatments and cool mist tent. Discontinue aerosolized racemic epinephrine per protocol. Monitor and reevaluate (within 1 hour). If clinical data remains the same, will recommend discharge.

Discussion

This case is instructive in that it reminds us just how sick children can be and how quickly they respond to intelligent therapy. The use of cool mist and decongestant aerosols for this patient, along with appropriate oxygen therapy, clearly prevented the necessity for intubation.

In the *second SOAP evaluation,* therapists who select to recommend intubation cannot be faulted. Many physicians would elect to do so at this juncture unless they, as we, feel that persistence and time are often great healers in this condition. Clearly, close monitoring at this juncture is indicated if the child is doing worse.

Finally, the fact that the patient was not dyspneic and no longer had stridor or retractions and that apical pulse was 89, respiratory rate was 15, blood pressure was 125/80, oxygen saturation was 97%, and breath sounds were normal should be translated directly to the assessment note in the *third SOAP evaluation*, even though the patient is improving and well on his way to recovery.

CHAPTER **8** Pneumonia

RESPONSE 1

S: Patient states he is very short of breath.

O: Vital signs: BP 165/90, HR 120, RR 33, T 39.5° C (103° F). Cough: frequent, strong, hacking, productive of small amount of white and yellow sputum. Skin: pale and damp. Over right lower lobe, increased tactile and vocal fremitus, dull percussion note, bronchial breath sounds. Spo_2: 92%. ABGs (on 2 L/min O_2 nc): pH 7.56, $Paco_2$ 24, HCO_3^- 22, Pao_2 56. CXR: Right lower lung lobe infiltrate, air bronchograms, and alveolar consolidation. WBC 21,000.

A: • Respiratory distress (vital signs, ABGs)
• Right lower lobe pneumonia: consolidation (fever, fremitus, percussion notes, bronchial breath sounds, and CXR)
• Bronchial secretions: infection likely (white and yellow sputum)
 • Good ability to mobilize bronchial secretions (strong cough)
• Acute alveolar hyperventilation with mild hypoxemia (ABGs)

P: Bronchial hygiene therapy per protocol (e.g., cough and deep breathing). Also obtain sputum for Gram stain and culture—induce if necessary. Trial period of hyperinflation therapy per protocol. Oxygen therapy per protocol. Monitor and reevaluate.

RESPONSE 2

S: "I feel worse than when I came in."

O: Vital signs: BP 140/70, HR 125, RR 35 and shallow, T 38.9° C (102° F). Strong, barking cough. Producing small amount of blood-streaked sputum. Cyanosis. Over right lower and middle lung lobes and left lower lobe, increased tactile and vocal fremitus, dull percussion notes, bronchial breath sounds, and crackles. Spo_2: 91%. ABGs: pH 7.55, $Paco_2$ 26, HCO_3^- 24, Pao_2 53.

A: • Continued respiratory distress (vital signs, ABGs)
• Alveolar consolidation or atelectasis likely in right lower and middle lobes and left lower lobe—condition possibly worsening (percussion notes and breath sounds, crackles)
• Bronchial secretions: small amount (sputum production)
• Acute alveolar hyperventilation with moderate hypoxemia—essentially unchanged (ABGs)

P: Up-date physician on patient's respiratory status. Continue bronchial hygiene therapy per protocol. Continue trial period of hyperinflation therapy per protocol. Up-regulate oxygen therapy per protocol. Monitor and reevaluate.

RESPONSE 3

S: "I'm breathing easier."

O: Vital signs: BP 135/85, HR 90, RR 19, T 37.3° C (99° F). Cough: strong and nonproductive. CXR: resolving pneumonia, consolidation or atelectasis in lower and middle right and lower left lobes. Increased tactile and vocal fremitus, dull percussion notes, and bronchial breath sounds. Spo_2: 97%. ABGs: pH 7.44, $Paco_2$ 35, HCO_3^- 24, Pao_2 163.

A: • Consolidation or atelectasis in right lower and middle and left lower lobes—resolving (CXR, chest assessment data)
• Normal acid-base status with overly corrected hypoxemia (ABGs).

P: Down-regulate or discontinue hyperinflation therapy at present intensity level. Continue to encourage cough and deep breathing. Down-regulate oxygen therapy per protocol. Reevaluate next shift. Check final results of sputum culture.

Discussion

This patient presents as a typical case of pneumonia with cough, fever, and signs of lobar consolidation. He has acute respiratory alkalosis secondary to hyperventilation. Initially the therapist should direct his attention to identifying the causative agent by inducing a sputum specimen for culture and to oxygenating the patient, presumably (in this case) with a low flow oxygen cannula.

Unfortunately there is no effective, specific respiratory care treatment modality for alveolar consolidation. Hyperinflation therapy may be of some benefit, especially when applied to partially consolidated alveoli. Just like any treatment modality, however, the effectiveness of the hyperinflation therapy must be assessed through the collection of objective data (e.g., arterial blood gases, chest x-ray films, or vital signs). It should also be noted that the response to oxygen therapy is often poor, since the patient almost certainly has a right-to-left intrapulmonary shunt across the pneumonic segment. It is hoped some ventilated and perfused alveoli will be able to pick up some of the deficit, but a degree of oxygen refractoriness should be expected when alveolar consolidation is present.

The patient is so hypoxemic, despite alveolar hyperventilation, that close monitoring obviously is necessary. Asking questions about the patient's alcoholism and pneumonia vaccine status are worthwhile and show the therapist is thinking beyond the immediate acute episode during his or her evaluation and treatment of the patient.

The *second assessment* reflects the fact that patients with pneumonia often feel worse when they are improving. The production of sputum is often seen as a worrisome event when actually it may herald the breaking up of the pneumonic infiltrate. Because the patient is still producing some sputum, bronchial hygiene therapy should be continued. The patient's Pao_2 has really not improved significantly, and a trial of a higher concentration of oxygen by Venturi or nonrebreathing oxygen mask may be helpful at this point. Improved oxygenation would help allay the patient's anxiety as well as that of the physician and treating therapist!

The *third assessment* shows that the patient is clearly improving. Down-regulation of the oxygen therapy toward room air is all that remains for the therapist to do. Ordinarily hyperinflation therapy would be reduced or discontinued at this time in preparation for an early discharge. The reader should recognize that the average length of stay for patients with pneumonia in an American hospital today is approximately 4 days. Such patients will leave the hospital with a resolving, but not completely cleared, pneumonic process. Improvement in the patient's clinical status and resolution of fever, dyspnea, and signs of toxicity, however, can and should be expected in this short period unless complications such as bacteremia, abscess, or empyema arise. Attention to what precipitated the admission is worthwhile, and review of the situation and recollection that this patient is a problem drinker would be appropriate before discharge, when attempts to interdict this process might be most helpful.

•• KEY POINT ANSWERS *For Pneumonia (DRG 89)*

1. Basic Concept Formation
   a. *No.* It is usually caused by an acute exposure to a sometimes contagious infectious agent. Identification of the precise causative infectious agent is helpful, as it allows specific (targeted) antibiotic therapy.
   b. *Yes.* The cough is not always productive, and obtaining a sputum specimen (see 1.a) is one of the *first tasks* of the RCP dealing with this condition.
   c. *Antibiotics* are used in *all* bacterial pneumonias and in a few viral pneumonias.
   d. *Yes.* In the United States, pneumonia is the sixth leading cause of death and the number 1 cause of death from infectious disease. One fifth of the estimated 4 million U.S. cases per year require hospitalization. The overall mortality of community acquired pneumonia (CAP) is 1% to 5%, but it may reach 25% in certain segments of the population (see 2.b).

2. Data Base Formation
   a. Pneumonia usually is an acute disease characterized by alveolar filling, called *consolidation,* in most bacterial pneumonias* and by *interstitial infiltration and thickening* in many viral pneumonias.
   b. Different bacteria and viruses are *responsible* for pneumonia in different segments of the population:
      (1) Chronic obstructive pulmonary disease (COPD) patients: *Streptococcus pneumoniae, Haemophilus influenzae,* and *Moraxella catarrhalis* (previously known as *Branhamella catarrhalis*).
      (2) Cystic fibrosis patients: *Pseudoumonas* and staphylococci.
      (3) Viral pneumonia patients: Prone to bacterial superinfection with *S. pneumoniae, H. influenzae,* and *Staphylococcus aureus.*
      (4) Nursing home patients: Methicillin-resistant *S. aureus, Mycobacterium tuberculosis,* gram-negative bacilli, respiratory syncytial virus (RSV), adenovirus, influenza virus.
      (5) Alcoholics: Aspiration pneumonia caused by oral or gastrointestinal flora (often with anaerobic organisms).
   c. The *main pathophysiologic mechanisms* activated by infectious alveolar consolidation (pneumonia) are the *immune response, shunt physiology, and decreased lung compliance* (see Fig. 1-5). In acute interstitial pneumonia, *alveolar-capillary diffusion block* is present, and the lung demonstrates stiffness or reduced compliance (see Fig. 1-6).
   d. *Severe* CAP is defined by the presence of one or more of the following clinical findings:
      (1) Respiratory frequency >30 breaths per minute
      (2) Pao_2/Fio_2 ratio <25 mm Hg
      (3) Requirement of mechanical ventilation
      (4) Involvement of multiple lobes or an increase in the size of the opacity by 50%
      (5) Shock: systolic BP <90 mm Hg, diastolic BP <60 mm Hg
      (6) Vasopressor required for more than 4 hours
      (7) Urine output <20 ml/h, or <50 ml/4 h
      (8) Acute renal failure requiring dialysis
   e. Criteria for consideration of *hospitalization* of CAP patients include the following:
      (1) Respiratory distress
      (2) High fever
      (3) Hypotension (systolic BP <100)
      (4) Altered mental status
      (5) Suppurative or metastatic infection
      (6) Significant coexisting disease
      (7) Severe laboratory abnormalities, that is, metabolic acidosis, elevated BUN and serum creatinine levels, hypernatremia >155 mmol/L.
   f. The *goals of therapy* in pneumonia, along with use of appropriate systemic antibiotics, are
      (1) Prevention (with pneumococcal or influenza vaccine) when appropriate
      (2) Fever control
      (3) Dyspnea control

---

*See color plate 9 in Des Jardins T, Burton GG: *Clinical manifestations & assessment of respiratory disease,* ed 3, St. Louis, 1995, Mosby.

(4) Relief of hypoxemia

(5) Clearance of airway secretions if present

(6) Ventilatory support if necessary

g. *Oxygen Therapy Protocol* (see box, p. 6) in all hypoxemic patients; *Bronchial Hygiene Therapy Protocol* in patients with excessive, poorly mobilized secretions (in the resolution phase of pneumonia); *ventilatory support* in the presence of acute ventilatory failure.

h. *Empyema, pleural effusion, involvement of other lobes, septicemia,* and *ventilatory failure* are complications of pneumonia.

3. Assessment

a. *Yes.* The patient reported fever, chills, and cough. He demonstrated respiratory distress, tachycardia, physical and x-ray findings indicating alveolar consolidation, and oxygen-resistant hypoxemia despite alveolar hyperventilation.

b. *Yes.* His *reduced ventilation-perfusion ratio* and *relative shunt physiology was evidenced in oxygen-refractory hypoxemia.* His alveolar consolidation resulted in *decreased lung compliance,* evidenced on chest physical examination by shallow, rapid breathing, and findings of alveolar consolidation on the admission chest x-ray film. His *immune response* was evidenced by his fever and elevated white blood cell count.

c. Initially, only his *respiratory rate* of 33/min. At the *second assessment* the pneumonic process apparent in *additional lobes* reflected the condition's severity.

4. Application

a. Sputum sample/induction **was** indicated because the patient was expectorating yellowish sputum. If the RCP did not think to "catch" some sputum when it was available, he or she *could* elect to induce it.

b. Oxygen therapy **was** indicated to try to relieve the patient's modest, but real, hypoxemia.

c. Bronchial hygiene **was** initially indicated, since the patient had some secretions. Encouragement of cough and deep breathing was initially appropriate. Failure to recognize this costs American hospitals millions of dollars each year.

d. Bronchodilator therapy **was not** indicated because pneumonia is primarily an anatomic alteration of the alveoli.

e. Hyperinflation therapy **was** indicated because there was evidence of atelectasis (pulmonary infiltrate). For example, a trial of incentive spirometry to prevent or treat any coincident atelectasis *may* have been appropriate. The therapeutic effect of hyperinflation therapy for consolidation is often disappointing. However, a trial period may be worth the effort.

5. Evaluation

a. The following results are to be expected:

(1) *Sputum induction:* expect to induce a satisfactory sputum sample promptly.

(2) *Oxygen therapy:* expect to modestly, but not totally, improve the patient's hypoxemia. The degree of success is inversely proportional to the degree of absolute shunt present. Improving the patient's hypoxemia may improve his dyspnea.

(3) *Bronchial hygiene:* expect to loosen secretions and to keep airways clear. Also works to prevent mucus plugging and atelectasis.

(4) *Hyperinflation therapy:* expect to offset the development of atelectasis and to improve oxygenation.

b. *Pulse oximetry* would be helpful to monitor the patient's hypoxemia. Follow-up ABGs and chest x-ray films are appropriate.

c. *Oxygen therapy* can be increased to an F_{IO_2} of 1.0. If this is not sufficient, the patient could be intubated and placed on an F_{IO_2} of 0.8 to 1.0, and a PEEP trial attempted. Severe pneumonia may improve with this approach, but it was not indicated here.

d. Consider *intubation* as in 5.c above.

6. Boundary Awareness

a. *Pulse oximetry and ABG analysis* are the best means to assess improvement. *Lysis of fever* often signals improvement; *recurrent fever* is often a sign of bacterial or viral superinfection. It is not unusual for the chest x-ray film to worsen initially after patient hydration has been achieved and parenteral antibiotics given. However, in severe CAP, extension of the infiltrate on the chest x-ray film may be an ominous sign.

b. *No,* not necessarily, if you are comfortable with the patient's lack of severity indicators.

c. Probably not at all. The patient was demonstrating continued improvement in fever and ABGs by the time of the *third assessment.*

d. *Ventilatory failure* was never an issue, as his Pa_{CO_2} was never elevated and his Pa_{O_2} was stable or improving.

CHAPTER 9 Acquired Immunodeficiency Syndrome (AIDS)

RESPONSE 1

S: "Sore throat and extremely irritating, nonproductive cough."

O: Cough: frequent, strong, and nonproductive. Neck: swollen lymph nodes. Vital signs: BP 137/90, HR 95, RR 20, T 37° C (98.6° F). Lung bases: dull percussion notes and bronchial breath sounds. CXR: infiltrates in lung bases (possible pneumonia). ABGs (room air): pH 7.47, $Paco_2$ 33, HCO_3^- 23, Pao_2 76.

A: • Increased work of breathing (general appearance, vital signs, ABGs)
• Alveolar consolidation (pneumonia) in lung bases (CXR, bronchial breath sounds, dull percussion notes)
• Acute alveolar hyperventilation with mild hypoxemia (ABGs)

P: Oxygenation therapy per protocol. Hyperinflation therapy per protocol (e.g., cough and deep breathe); try to obtain sputum for Gram stain and culture. Monitor and reevaluate.

RESPONSE 2

S: "I'm not breathing very well. I'm getting worse."

O: Cough: frequent, strong, and nonproductive. Vital signs: BP 185/100, HR 125, RR 31, T normal. RML, RLL, and LLL: dull percussion notes and bronchial breath sounds. Spo_2: 92%. ABGs: pH 7.54, $Paco_2$ 27, HCO_3^- 22, Pao_2 54.

A: • Continued increased work of breathing (general appearance, vital signs, ABGs)
• Alveolar consolidation in lung bases (earlier CXR and present bronchial breath sounds, dull percussion notes)
• Acute alveolar hyperventilation with worsening hypoxemia (ABGs)
• Possible impending ventilatory failure

P: Up-regulate oxygenation therapy per protocol. Up-regulate hyperinflation therapy per protocol. Contact physician and discuss present respiratory status; request a repeat CXR; consider diagnostic/therapeutic bronchoscopy if CXR is worse. Monitor and reevaluate.

RESPONSE 3

S: The patient made a head gesture that he was doing poorly.

O: No cough noted. Vital signs: BP 170/85, HR 145, RR 30 and shallow, T 40° C (104° F). Dull percussion notes and bronchial breath sounds over RML, RLL, and LLL. CXR: greater density and air bronchograms: RML, RLL, and LLL. Spo_2: 77%. ABGs: pH 7.28, $Paco_2$ 61, HCO_3^- 27, Pao_2 47.

A: • Continued increased work of breathing (general appearance, vital signs, ABGs)
• Alveolar consolidation in RML, RLL, LLL worsening (CXR, bronchial breath sounds, dull percussion notes)
• Acute ventilatory failure with severe hypoxemia (ABGs)

P: Contact physician stat: Recommend mechanical ventilation, transfer to intensive care unit (ICU), and bronchscopy. Up-regulate oxygenation therapy per protocol. Up-regulate hyperinflation therapy per protocol. Monitor and reevaluate.

Discussion

This case presents as an undiagnosed pulmonary infiltrate of uncertain duration. A history of irritating cough in an intravenous drug user and a pneumonic infiltrate on chest x-ray film should raise all sorts of red flags with the medical team. In this case it clearly did not. On admission his blood gases were not severely abnormal, although they showed mild resting hypoxemia despite alveolar hyperventilation. It appears that he was admitted largely on the basis of the chest x-ray film. At this point many clinicians would have elected to simply treat him as an outpatient with antibiotics and to follow him in the clinic or office.

After the patient was admitted, he rapidly progressed to acute ventilatory failure with severe hypoxemia over the next 4 days. His chest x-ray film and blood gases became worse, his dyspnea became more severe, and he became acutely febrile.

Note that 3 days into his hospitalization a diagnostic/therapeutic bronchoscopy was suggested in Response 2. This was suggested basically because no cause for the pneumonia had been demonstrated. Also note that on the second assessment the patient's blood gases were significantly abnormal. Specifically, his Pao_2 had fallen from 76 to 54 mm Hg, despite the fact that the second blood gas was obtained, presumably, on a higher Fio_2 (the increase is assumed from Response 1). Calculation shows an enormous difference in the probable alveolar-arterial oxygen gradient between these two blood gases. The plan developed on the second evaluation suggests again that there is really little that the treating therapist can do for pneumonia per se. Basically he or she can attempt to oxygenate the patient, control airway secretions, and make sure (to the best of his or her ability) that the cause of the pneumonia is identified.

On the *final evaluation* the medical team is becoming concerned that the patient may have acquired immunodeficiency syndrome (AIDS), and appropriate blood work is ordered. The therapist knows that what *he* is treating is the *complication* of that syndrome, specifically the pneumonic infiltrate. He must help assure that appropriate biopsies and cultures are sent off once a bronchoscopy is performed (after the patient is on a ventilator). Because about 80% of acute, progressive pneumonias in patients testing positive for the human immunodeficiency virus (HIV) are caused by *Pneumocystis carinii* pneumonia (PCP), the therapist should assure that special stains (Giemsa and silver methenamine) for PCP are performed in a timely manner.

Finally, in the last evaluation the reader should have been aware that the patient had severe shunt physiology (severe refractory hypoxemia despite supplemental oxygen therapy) and acute ventilatory failure. The hypoxemia alone is enough to suggest to the therapist that the patient is approaching dangerous boundaries and that a stat call to the attending physician is indicated. Clearly, in the last evaluation, intubation, ventilatory support, and positive end-expiratory pressure are almost certainly mandatory unless a "no-code" order is in effect per the patient's wishes.

CHAPTER **10**   Lung Abscess

RESPONSE 1

S: "I spit all the time."

O: Thin, undernourished, poor hygiene. Appears cyanotic. Frequent moderate-to-weak cough with foul smelling purulent sputum. Vital signs: BP 145/75, HR 110, RR 33, T 39.3° C (102.8° F). Right middle and lower lobes: tactile and vocal fremitus, crackles and rhonchi. ABGs (2 L/min nc): pH 7.49, $Paco_2$ 30, HCO_3^- 22, Pao_2 63. CXR: Partially fluid-filled, 10 cm cavity in RML and increased opacity in RML and RLL.

A: • Increased work of breathing (general appearance, vital signs, ABGs)
• Malnourished (inspection)
• Lung abscess (RML)—likely open to bronchus (CXR, sputum)
• Consolidation vs. atelectasis likely in RML and RLL (CXR: increased opacity)
• Excessive bronchial secretions (purulent sputum)
   • Moderate-to-weak cough
• Acute alveolar hyperventilation with mild-to-moderate hypoxemia.

P: Oxygen therapy per protocol. Hyperinflation therapy per protocol. Bronchial hygiene therapy per protocol (check blood and sputum, culture and sensitivity). Suggest nutrition consult. Monitor and reevaluate.

RESPONSE 2

S: "I'm not as short of breath as yesterday."

O: Alert and oriented. Cyanotic. Frequent and weak cough. Sputum: thick and purulent. Vital signs: BP 135/80, HR 98, RR 20, T 37.9° C (100.2° F). RML and RLL tactile and vocal fremitus, crackles and rhonchi. ABGs: pH 7.48, $Paco_2$ 34, HCO_3^- 23, Pao_2 81. Spo_2: 96%.

A: • Continued respiratory distress (vital signs, ABGs)
• Abscess (RML) likely open to bronchus (CXR, sputum)
• Consolidation or atelectasis likely in RML and RLL (CXR: increased opacity)
• Excessive bronchial secretions (thick and purulent sputum)
• Poor ability to mobilize secretions (weak cough)
• Acute alveolar hyperventilation with corrected hypoxemia (ABGs)

P: Maintain oxygenation therapy intensity per protocol. Up-regulate bronchial hygiene therapy per protocol. Maintain hyperinflation therapy per protocol. Monitor and reevaluate.

RESPONSE 3

S: "You doctors cured my d . . . cough."

O: Skin: normal color. No spontaneous cough. Can produce a strong cough upon request. No sputum noted. Vital signs: BP 127/82, HR 86, RR 16, T normal. Crackles over the RLL. ABGs: pH 7.43, $Paco_2$ 36, HCO_3^- 24, Pao_2 163. Spo_2: 97%.

A: • Abscess (RML): improved (CXR, no sputum)
• Consolidation and atelectasis still likely in RML (CXR: persistent infiltrate)
• Normal acid-base status with overly corrected hypoxemia (ABGs)

P: Down-regulate oxygenation therapy per protocol. Down-regulate or discontinue bronchial hygiene therapy per protocol. Maintain hyperinflation therapy per protocol (e.g., 24 to 48 hours). Monitor and reevaluate daily until discharge.

Discussion

Production of foul smelling, putrid, yellow-green sputum should immediately raise at least three diagnostic possibilities in the mind of the respiratory care practitioner: lung abscess, bronchiectasis, or communicating empyema. The fact that the patient had carious teeth and a vagrant lifestyle should be enough to make the diagnosis of lung abscess almost without a chest x-ray film. At any rate, it is clear that the patient is acutely ill and febrile upon arrival at the hospital and has localized findings in the right lung. Furthermore the patient is moderately hypoxemic despite alveolar hyperventilation and is chronically malnourished.

The initial plan to oxygenate the patient, to institute bronchial hygiene, and to suggest nutrition evaluation is entirely appropriate. Since the patient has had a clear change in mentation and is now confused, a toxic drug and alcohol blood screen is an excellent idea. The patient's course within the next few days will depend largely on mentation being clear so that she may cooperate with the chest physical therapy procedures. It would be tragic to miss a toxic drug level of barbiturates, cocaine, or other sedatives. The patient's alcohol consumption history speaks for itself. Finally, the possibility of a head injury (due to street lifestyle) cannot be ruled out. The reader who noted the confusion of the patient and said so in the subjective or objective analysis is to be congratulated.

The benefit of hyperinflation therapy may be marginal in this case. Infiltates coincident with a lung cavity are almost certainly pneumonic. Consolidated alveoli may not respond at all to lung expansion therapy. However, because atelectasis was also a possibility, a trial period of hyperinflation therapy was certainly warranted in this case.

At the time of the *second assessment* the patient's oxygenation is clearly being well served by her current oxygen and bronchial hygiene therapy. It is now time to check the laboratory to see if sputum and blood cultures have been productive; in which case, antibiotic therapy would need to be continued or regulated appropriately. In patients with infectious lung disease, it is the *therapist's responsibility* to have this information available for the treating physician as soon as possible.

The *final assessment* indicates that the patient has clearly improved. This should be reflected in the therapist's assessment notes. The sequence of events necessitating this admission could probably be prevented in the future. This could well be mentioned in the final treatment plan.

CHAPTER **11** Tuberculosis

RESPONSE 1

S: "I can't get my breath."

O: Cyanotic, malnourished, weak, and in obvious respiratory distress. Cough: frequent, moderate amount of yellow sputum mixed with fresh blood, history of previous expectoration of blood. Vital signs: BP 170/95, HR 110, RR 26, T 38.3° C (101° F). Dull percussion notes, increased tactile and vocal fremitus, and bronchial breath sounds over the right and left lung bases. Crackles and rhonchi in RUL. Pleural friction rub: RLL between the 5th and 6th ribs in the anterior axillary line. CXR: LLL, RML, and RUL, increased opacity consistent with pneumonia. 5 cm cavity in LUL. ABGs (room air): pH 7.53, Pa_{CO_2} 51, HCO_3^- 41, Pa_{O_2} 50. COHb: 8.5 vol%. Sp_{O_2}: 88%.

A:
 • Respiratory distress (general appearance, vital signs, ABGs)
 • Alveolar consolidation or atelectasis: LLL, RML, RUL (dull percussion notes, bronchial breath sounds, CXR)
 • Excessive bronchial secretions and hemoptysis (sputum production, rhonchi)
   • Infection likely (yellow sputum)
   • Effective cough (strong)
   • Cavity LUL (CXR): probably tuberculous
 • Acute alveolar hyperventilation superimposed on chronic ventilatory failure with moderate hypoxemia (history, ABGs, CXR)
   • Sp_{O_2} misleading because of COHb

P: Oxygenation therapy per protocol. Bronchial hygiene therapy per protocol, for example, chest physical therapy over left upper lobe to enhance drainage of cavity. Sputum culture. Hyperinflation therapy per protocol. Monitor and reevaluate.

RESPONSE 2

S: "My cough is a lot better."

O: Positive tuberculin reaction. PFT: moderate-to-severe restrictive disorder. CXR: improved opacity of lung bases. Improved cyanosis and respiratory distress. Cough: frequent and productive of small amount of opaque sputum. Vital signs: BP 143/90, HR 92, RR 18, T 37.4° C (99.3° F). Dull percussion notes and bronchial breath sounds over lung bases. Rhonchi over RML, not so intense as on admission. ABGs: pH 7.48, Pa_{CO_2} 60, HCO_3^- 42, Pa_{O_2} 61. Sp_{O_2}: 91%.

A:
 • Continued respiratory distress, but improving (vital signs, ABGs)
 • Tuberculosis, likely (positive tuberculin reaction)
 • Alveolar consolidation or atelectasis, improving (history, CXR, dull percussion notes, bronchial breath sounds)
 • Excessive bronchial secretions in RML, improving (rhonchi)
 • Acute alveolar hyperventilation superimposed on chronic ventilatory failure with mild hypoxemia, improving (ABGs)

P: Up-regulate oxygenation therapy per protocol (careful not to knock out hypoxic drive to breathe). Continue bronchial hygiene therapy per protocol (present intensity appears to be adequate). Down-regulate or discontinue hyperinflation therapy per protocol (present cough efficiency appears to be adequate). Monitor and reevaluate.

RESPONSE 3

S: "I think I'm ready to run a marathon."

O: Skin: moderately pale and cyanotic. Respiratory distress no longer present. No spontaneous, uncontrolled cough noted. Strong, nonproductive cough on request. Vital signs: BP 135/85, HR 80, RR 10, T 37° C (98.6° F). Palpation and percussion: negative. Normal vesicular breath sounds in lower lung fields. ABGs (on 1 L/min O_2 nc): pH 7.42, $Paco_2$ 72, HCO_3^- 45, Pao_2 78. Spo_2: 94%.

A: • Tuberculosis; likely (positive tuberculin reaction and acid-fast sputum stains)
  • Chronic ventilatory failure with mild or corrected hypoxemia: normal for this patient (current ABGs, compared to out-patient baseline 6 months earlier)

P: Discontinue oxygenation therapy per protocol. Continue bronchial hygiene therapy per protocol. Discontinue hyperinflation therapy per protocol (if have not done so already). Discuss pulmonary rehabilitation and education with patient (if possible) and staff at the Samaritan Shelter. Consider smoking cessation.

Discussion

The last decade of the twentieth century has seen a disconcerting rise in the number of active cases of tuberculosis, particularly among the poor, the homeless, those living in crowded urban settings, and those with various degrees of immune suppression. The presentation of a homeless, alcoholic patient with cough, fever, and hemoptysis is, of course, highly suggestive of tuberculosis.

A chest x-ray film that shows a pneumonic infiltrate with cavity formation nearly makes the diagnosis, long before the results of the sputum acid fast smear and tuberculin skin test are in hand. Most clinical cases of tuberculosis are not associated with gas exchange difficulties; however, the fact that this patient presented with cyanosis, hypoxemia, a degree of CO_2 retention, and more than a few pulmonary infiltrates suggests that pulmonary tuberculosis may be only one of his respiratory diagnoses.

Note that in the *first assessment* the patient had significant carboxyhemoglobinemia; thus his saturation when corrected for his carbon monoxide level was considerably lower than the pulse oximetry determined hemoglobin saturation of 88% (in truth, 88 − 8.5 = 79.5%). Also note in the first assessment that the therapist picked up on the patient's secretions and history of smoking and placed him on a vigorous program of bronchial hygiene. This could consist of metered dose inhaler (MDI)–administered bronchodilators, and mucolytics if indicated. Treatment should be aggressive at first, since the patient was complaining of respiratory distress. Because of the finding of a cavity in an undiagnosed patient, careful chest physical therapy with percussion and postural drainage to that area of the lung was indicated.

The patient's hypoxemia could probably be treated with low flow oxygen therapy with careful monitoring of subsequent blood gases to be sure that CO_2 retention did not develop. The use of hyperinflation therapy at the end of the first assessment is debatable, since the patient was successfully clearing secretions.

It should also be noted that in the handling of the first part of this case the patient was not properly isolated given the history and x-ray findings. Another caveat is that the bronchoscopic secretions were appropriately examined for malignant cells as well as for routine and acid fast organisms (the first because of the patient's cigarette smoking history and the second because of the by then recognized probability that the staff would be dealing here with active tuberculosis).

A final caveat is that if possible the patient should enter a good rehabilitation program where smoking cessation and nutrition counseling are readily available. Because his blood gases were so borderline, rechecking them while he was an out-patient on low flow oxygen was certainly indicated.

CHAPTER **12** Fungal Diseases of the Lungs

RESPONSE 1

S: "I feel short of breath, and my joints are swollen and painful."

O: Cyanotic. Cough: frequent and strong, producing moderate amounts of thick, yellow sputum. Vital signs: BP 160/90, HR 93, RR 18, T 37.8° C (100° F). Palpation: red lesions on anterior chest and left cheek. Auscultation: Bilateral crackles and rhonchi in lung bases. CXR: Bilateral fibrosis and calcification and spherical nodules. Two to three, 1- to 3-cm cavities in both upper lobes. ABGs (room air): pH 7.51, $Paco_2$ 29, HCO_3^- 22, Pao_2 64.

A: • Moderate respiratory distress (cyanosis, vital signs)
 • Excessive amounts of thick, yellow bronchial secretions (sputum, rhonchi)
  • Infection likely (yellow sputum)
 • Alveolar fibrosis and calcification and cavities (CXR)
 • Acute alveolar hyperventilation with mild hypoxemia (ABGs)

P: Oxygen therapy per protocol. Bronchial hygiene therapy per protocol. Sputum culture. Monitor and reevaluate (e.g., q6-8h).

RESPONSE 2

S: "I still can't get a good breath of air."

O: Respiratory distress: cyanotic, short of breath. Positive spherulin skin test. Coccidioidomycosis organisms seen in sputum smear. Frequent strong cough: moderate amount of thick, opaque sputum. Vital signs: BP 165/95, HR 97, RR 24, T normal. Bilateral crackles and rhonchi in the lung bases. Spo_2: 88%. ABGs: pH 7.54, $Paco_2$ 27, HCO_3^- 21, Pao_2 55.

A: • Coccidioidomycosis (positive spherulin skin test, sputum smear)
 • Continued respiratory distress (cyanosis, vital signs)
 • Excessive amounts of thick bronchial secretions (sputum, rhonchi)
 • Acute alveolar hyperventilation with moderate hypoxemia (ABGs)

P: Up-regulate oxygen therapy per protocol. Continue bronchial hygiene therapy per protocol. Monitor and reevaluate (e.g., q4-6h). Suggest repeat CXR.

RESPONSE 3

S: "I'm breathing much better."

O: No obvious respiratory distress. No spontaneous cough. Strong, nonproductive cough on request. Vital signs: BP 135/88, HR 80, RR 14, T normal. Bilateral crackles in the lung bases. Spo_2: 91%. ABGs: pH 7.44, $Paco_2$ 34, HCO_3^- 23, Pao_2 71.

A: • Adequate bronchial hygiene status (nonproductive cough, absence of rhonchi, crackles expected in lung fibrosis)
 • Normal acid-base status with mild hypoxemia (ABGs)

P: Down-regulate or discontinue oxygen therapy per protocol (Pao_2 of 71 may be the patient's personal best). Discontinue bronchial hygiene therapy per protocol. Monitor and reevaluate (e.g., q24h).

Discussion

Respiratory care practitioners (RCPs) who work in the Southwest where coccidioidomycosis is endemic would probably anticipate the diagnosis in the patient with bilateral pulmonary infiltrates, swollen tender joints, and the typical skin rash of this lesion. Others could not be blamed if they missed this fact until the coccidioidal skin test came back positive and the sputum fungal smear demonstrated the coccidioidomycosis organism.

The *first assessment,* that the patient is hypoxemic despite alveolar hyperventilation and that he has alveolar fibrosis and cavity formation, is correct. For the hypoxemia, oxygen therapy is appropriate and should be started with a nasal oxygen cannula at 1 to 2 L/min and then regulated with a pulse oximeter. In treating this case as any other pneumonia, the assessing RCP should quickly obtain a sputum, Gram stain, and acid fast bacillus and fungal preparations, and this was appropriately done here. The treating RCP would do well to understand the use of tuberculin and fungal testing in such patients and to understand, as in other pneumonic infiltrates, that his or her impact here once that is done would probably be minimal.

In the *second assessment,* 4 days later, the offending organism has been isolated and appropriate therapy with intravenous amphotericin-B started. The patient continues to be hypoxemic, and up-regulation of his oxygen therapy (perhaps to 3 or 4 L/min, or with a nonrebreathing mask if that is not successful) is indicated. Because the patient is still coughing up thick, opaque sputum and because his dyspnea is not relieved so far, up-regulation of bronchial hygiene program with a trial of bronchodilator therapy and mucolytic therapy might well be in order. Because the patient is not improving, a repeat chest x-ray film appears indicated.

At the *last assessment,* 10 days after the patient's admission to the hospital, clear improvement is noted. Oximetry reveals good peripheral oxygen saturation, and the blood gases are much improved. Now is the time for the treating therapist to reduce the intensity of the patient's respiratory care, and this is illustrated in the appropriate response for this section of the case study.

CHAPTER **13**   Pulmonary Edema

RESPONSE 1

S: "I don't think I'm having a serious problem."

O: Vital signs: BP 175/130, HR 145 and irregular, RR 22. Anxious. Cough: small amount of frothy, pink secretions. Bilateral, dull percussion notes over the lower lung areas. Bilateral inspiratory crackles and expiratory wheezes over the lower lobes. ABGs (2 L/min O_2 nc): pH 7.56, $Paco_2$ 28, HCO_3^- 20, Pao_2 61. CXR: dense, fluffy opacities in lower lungs; left cardiac enlargement.

A: • Respiratory distress (vital signs, ABGs)
   • Hypertension (blood pressure)
   • Acute pulmonary edema (crackles, distended neck veins, CXR)
   • Acute alveolar hyperventilation with moderate hypoxemia (ABGs)
   • Small airway secretions, alveolar flooding, interstitial edema or any combination of these (crackles)
   • Bronchospasm?? (wheezing most likely caused by airway secretions)

P: Oxygen therapy per protocol. Hyperinflation therapy per protocol (e.g., continuous positive airway pressure [CPAP]). May consider bronchodilator therapy if wheezing is still present at next SOAP. Monitor and reevaluate (vital signs, pulse oximetry, ABGs, cardiac enzymes).

RESPONSE 2

S: "I still don't feel great."

O: Vital signs: BP 160/125, HR 105 and regular, RR 20. Slight improvement in cyanosis. Distended neck veins persist. Urine output: 650 ml. Frequent, nonproductive cough. Bilateral inspiratory crackles and expiratory wheezes over lower lobes. Spo_2: 84%. ABGs: pH 7.54, $Paco_2$ 25, HCO_3^- 18, Pao_2 51.

A: • Continued respiratory distress (vital signs, ABGs)
   • Persistent acute pulmonary edema (physical findings, CXR)
   • Worsening acute alveolar hyperventilation with moderate hypoxemia (more severe than admission) (ABGs)
   • Small airway secretions (crackles)
   • Bronchospasm?? (wheezing most likely caused by airway secretions)

P: Up-regulate oxygen therapy per protocol. Up-regulate hyperinflation therapy per protocol (e.g., mask CPAP). Trial period of bronchodilator therapy per protocol. Continue to monitor and reevaluate (vital signs, pulse oximetry, ABGs).

RESPONSE 3

S: "I'm breathing easier."

O: Vital signs: BP 140/115, HR 95 and regular, RR 16. No longer cyanotic. Urine output: 850 ml over past 2 hours. Neck veins no longer distended. Cough: strong, nonproductive. Bilateral crackles over lower lobes. Spo_2: 97%. ABGs: pH 7.44, $Paco_2$ 36, HCO_3^- 24, Pao_2 190.

A: • Pulmonary edema (history and physical findings)
   • Condition appears to be improving
   • Small airway secretions (crackles)
   • Normal ventilatory/acid-base status with overly corrected hypoxemia (ABGs)

P: Reduce hyperinflation therapy per protocol. Down-regulate oxygen therapy per protocol. Discontinue bronchodilator therapy. Continue to monitior and reevaluate (vital signs, pulse oximetry, ABGs).

Discussion

The patient's presentation with a known cardiac history, cough productive of foamy, pink-tinged sputum, neck vein distension, peripheral edema, and rapid atrial fibrillation are virtually pathognomonic of acute pulmonary edema. The therapist should be aware that the following conditions may precipitate pulmonary edema in a given patient: (1) acute myocardial infarction, (2) hypertension, (3) valvular heart disease, (4) rapid ventricular rate with inadequate filling time of atria and ventricles, and (5) exogenous fluid overload.

The treatment of this condition is oxygen therapy, maintenance of alveolar volume with positive end-expiratory pressure (PEEP) or CPAP therapy, and bronchial hygiene directed at mechanically removing secretions from the airway. In the past, ethanol has been added to the inspirate to "reduce surface tension of the bubbles in the secretions," but this is falling out of favor. Although trial periods may be appropriate, bronchodilator therapy typically is not required, since smooth muscle bronchospasm usually does not occur in this condition.

In the *first assessment* the therapist may well have mentioned his interest in cardiac enzymes, since treatment of the patient with acute myocardial infarction causing pulmonary edema is somewhat different than that of the other conditions mentioned above.

After the *second SOAP* the patient is clearly not doing well, his Pa_{O_2} is still low, and now the question of a coincident metabolic acidosis arises. This is not uncommon in patients with cardiac disease who may be hypotensive. The blood gas observed here is more worrisome, since the Pa_{O_2} is low despite alveolar hyperventilation. If the patient were not tolerating mask CPAP, intubation for intervention of PEEP therapy would be indicated at this point. If the patient were not already in the ICU, we would transfer him there about now.

After the *third SOAP* this case highlights the rapid therapeutic response that can occur in most patients with pulmonary edema. Even patients with acute myocardial infarction as the cause of their pulmonary edema generally improve rapidly with therapy such as that outlined here. The cardiac inotropic and chronotropic agents and the intravenous diuretic therapy started in the emergency room 9 hours or so ago have now exerted their maximum effect. If monitoring of pulse oximetry and blood gases in the next 24 hours continued to give reassuring results, the therapist could probably sign off of this case and the patient can go on his trip.

•◆ KEY POINT ANSWERS   **For Pulmonary Edema (DRG 87)**

1. **Basic Concept Formation**
   a. **Yes.** When the pump action of the left heart fails, pulmonary venous drainage is impaired and first interstitial and then alveolar edema occur. The body perceives this through several mechanisms (see 2.b below) and responds with a sensation of dyspnea.
   b. The pulmonary venous pressure *increases* when the pump action of the left heart fails.
   c. The word *edema* comes from the Greek *oidema,* meaning swelling.
   d. *Smoking, obesity,* and *age* are common risk factors for both heart and lung disease.
2. **Data Base Formation**
   a. In mild or early pulmonary edema there is *alveolar-capillary membrane swelling* and thickening with edema fluid. In more advanced cases, *alveolar flooding* with edema fluid occurs.* This fluid may fill the airways up to the oropharynx, where it is clinically called *foaming pulmonary edema.* The reader may note similarities between this pathology and that of near drowning.†
   b. Increased alveolar-capillary membrane thickness results in alveolar diffusion blockade. The lung is stiff and waterlogged and demonstrates reduced compliance (see Fig. 1-6). Relative shunt physiology develops as alveolar flooding occurs. Hypoxemia drives various oxygen and pressure receptors, which increase heart rate and ventilatory rate. If the cardiac output is **not controlled** by intrinsic heart disease, cardiac output may increase.
   c. *(See 2.b above).* Vascular markings will increase, progressing to *"white out" of the chest x-ray film* as the pulmonary edema worsens. *Bronchial breath sounds* and *crackles* will be heard. *Restrictive pathology* will be observed on pulmonary function testing. *Hypoxemia* despite alveolar hyperventilation will be noted.
   d. *Chest pain, orthopnea, paroxysmal nocturnal dyspnea,* and *peripheral edema* are common signs and symptoms of congestive heart failure and of pulmonary edema. *Systemic hypertension* may be noted and indeed is a common cause of left ventricular failure. Various left-sided *cardiac murmurs* may reflect aortic or mitral valvular disease as the cause of the patient's pulmonary edema. *Gallop cardiac rhythms* may suggest *cardiomyopathy* as the cause of the heart failure. Signs of *hypothyroidism* may be a clue to myxedematous cardiomyopathy.
   e. The main goals of therapy are *reduction of pulmonary venous* and *left ventricular end-diastolic pressure, relief of dyspnea,* and *treatment of hypoxemia.* If *ventilatory failure* should occur, *support of alveolar ventilation* would be an additional goal.
   f. Following are standard TDPs that might achieve these goals:
      (1) Pharmacologic means are available to achieve the ends of reducing pulmonary venous hypertension and increased left ventricular end-diastolic pressure. These means are **not** in the standard respiratory care practitioner's armamentarium. They include antihypertensives, antiarrhythmic agents, diuretics, and cardiac inotropic and chronotropic agents. Their effects are evaluated in the acutely ill by *pulmonary artery (Swan-Ganz) catheter monitoring,* a task which **is** in the job description of many critical care, institutionally certified RCPs (see below).
      (2) The treatment of dyspnea in these patients is often difficult. *Oxygen Therapy Protocols* (see box, p. 6) are absolutely necessary and may sometimes only be effective when used with *CPAP* in *Hyperinflation Therapy Protocols* (see box, p. 6).
      (3) If ventilatory failure develops, mechanical ventilation therapy is used in conjunction with PEEP therapy in Hyperinflation Therapy Protocols (see box, p. 6).
   g. Following are the outcomes, adverse effects, and monitors of the preceding protocols:
      (1) The *outcomes* desired would be improvement in hypoxemia to Sao_2 >92% and treatment of acute ventilatory failure with early extubation should ventilatory management become necessary.
      (2) The only *adverse effect* worth noting in this selection of therapies is *barotrauma* secondary to high mean airway pressures.
      (3) Appropriate *monitors* in acute pulmonary edema include the following:
          (a) Spo_2

*See color plate 14 in Des Jardins T, Burton GG: *Clinical manifestations & assessment of respiratory disease,* ed. 3, St Louis, 1995, Mosby.
†See color plate 28 in Des Jardins T, Burton GG: *Clinical manifestations & assessment of respiratory disease,* ed. 3, St Louis, 1995, Mosby.

(b) ECG rate, rhythm, and morphology

(c) Intake and output records and daily weights

(d) Serial chest x-ray films

(e) Careful monitoring of mean airway pressure in ventilated patients

(f) Weaning parameters if extubation is contemplated

3. **Assessment**

a. *Yes.* He had a history of *hypertension, cigarette smoking,* and *atrial fibrillation* in the recent past.

b. *Yes.* He had tachycardia, atrial fibrillation with a rapid ventricular response, tachypnea, cyanosis, foamy, pink tracheal secretions, and severe peripheral edema. Auscultation of the chest revealed crackles. His chest x-ray film showed cardiomegaly and the centrally dense hilar infiltrates typical of the disorder.

c. *Yes.* His dyspnea reflected his *alveolar-capillary block and decreased lung compliance.*

d. Literally *all* the manifestations listed above indicate that he was severely, if not critically, ill.

4. **Application**

a. Oxygen therapy **was** indicated because of his *cardiac irritability* and significant *hypoxemia* despite alveolar hyperventilation. Morphine sulfate is often given for acute pulmonary edema. If the patient's hyperventilation were to stop as a result of such therapy, his Pao_2 would drop further.

b. *Monitoring* **was** indicated for *all* the reasons listed in answer 2.g above.

c. The use of *bronchial hygiene therapy* in this case **is open to debate.** He did have a "small" amount of secretions and wheezes on admission, and certainly *deep breathing and coughing* and p.r.n. *suctioning* would be appropriate then.

d. *Bronchodilators* must be used with caution in patients with cardiac disease. There were **no** clear indications.

e. *Hyperinflation therapy* **was** indicated to increase and stabilize alveolar size.

f. Mechanical ventilation **was not** indicated in this patient, as he tolerated the CPAP begun at the time of the *second assessment,* and CO_2 retention never developed.

5. **Evaluation**

a. Skillful oxygen and hyperinflation therapy should *improve hypoxemia and decrease the alveolar-arterial oxygen gradient.* The *heart rate and respiratory rate should fall.*

b. Look for *improvement in all monitors* discussed in 2.g above. Improvement in the chest x-ray film may lag behind improvement in static compliance and ABGs.

c. *Mask oxygen therapy* can be increased to an Fio_2 of 1.0. *Mask CPAP* tolerances vary, but 12-15 cm H_2O is at the upper limit of most individuals' tolerance. *PEEP pressures* in excess of 15 cm H_2O are associated with an increased risk of *barotrauma.*

d. *Mask or cannula oxygen therapy* is inexpensive and relatively safe (remote risk here of oxygen toxicity or hypoventilation). *Mask CPAP* is not well tolerated by most individuals but is certainly less invasive and less costly than intubation and *mechanical ventilation.* A *pulmonary artery catheter* carries the risk of infection, pneumothorax, arrhythmias, and embolization.

e. Therapy in *ventilated* patients with pulmonary edema could be reduced in the following order:

(1) Reduce PEEP pressures to 5 cm H_2O

(2) Wean from pressure support

(3) Extubate and put on mask Fio_2 5%-10% higher than ventilator Fio_2

(4) Titrate Fio_2

6. **Boundary Awareness**

a. His A-a oxygen gradient would worsen, and his *Pao_2 would fall.* His respiratory rate would *increase,* as would his *dyspnea.* His *weight would increase,* and he would be in *positive fluid balance.* His *chest x-ray* film would show increasing opacity.

b. If any of the above happen.

c. Before *intubation* of the patient.

d. The $Paco_2$ would rise, and *acute respiratory* (and possibly metabolic) *acidemia* would be seen.

e. See 5.d above.

CHAPTER **14** Pulmonary Embolism

S: "My breathing is okay."

O: No remarkable respiratory distress noted. Vital signs: BP 115/75, HR 75, RR 11. Tenderness over left shoulder and left anterior chest area. Normal vesicular breath sounds. CXR: normal. ABGs (partial rebreathing mask): pH 7.4, $Paco_2$ 41, HCO_3^- 24, Pao_2 504 mm Hg. Spo_2: 97%.

A: • No remarkable respiratory problems
• Normal acid-base status with overoxygenation

P: Discontinue or reduce oxygen therapy per protocol.

S: "I feel awful. I'm short of breath and lightheaded."

O: Cyanotic, agitated, and dyspneic. Cough produces small amount of blood-tinged sputum. Vital signs: BP 90/45, HR 125, RR 30, T normal. Slight wheezing throughout both lung fields. Pleural friction rub, right middle lobe. ECG: normal sinus rhythm, sinus tachycardia, atrial flutter. Hemodynamic indices: increased CVP, RAP, $\overline{PA}$, RVSWI, and PVR and a decreased PCWP, CO, SV, SVI, and CI. CXR: atelectasis and consolidation in the right middle lobe. ABGs: pH 7.53, $Paco_2$ 26, HCO_3^- 21 mmol/L, Pao_2 53 mm Hg. Spo_2: 89%.

A: • Hypotension (BP)
• Respiratory distress (cyanosis, heart rate, respiratory rate, ABGs)
• Pulmonary embolism and infarction likely (history, vital signs, CXR, ECG, blood-tinged sputum, wheezing, pleural friction rub)
• Bronchospasm, probably secondary to pulmonary embolism or infarction (wheezing)
• Alveolar atelectasis and consolidation (CXR)
• Acute alveolar hyperventilation with moderate hypoxemia (ABGs)
• Pulmonary artery hypertenstion and low cardiac output probably secondary to pulmonary embolism (clinical presentation and hemodynamic data)

P: Contact physician to request transfer to ICU. Oxygen therapy per protocol. Bronchodilator therapy per protocol. Monitor and reevaluate (e.g., in 30 minutes). Remain on standby with mechanical ventilator.

S: N/A (patient not responsive)

O: Ventilation-perfusion scan: no blood flow to the right middle lobe. Cyanotic. Cough: small amount of blood-tinged sputum. Vital signs: BP 70/35, HR 160, RR 25 and shallow. Palpation was negative. Dull percussion notes over the right middle lobe. Wheezing over both lung fields; pleural friction rub over the right middle lobe. ECG: alternates between a normal sinus rhythm, sinus tachycardia, and atrial flutter. Hemodynamic indices: increased CVP, RAP, $\overline{PA}$, RVSWI, and PVR and a decreased PCWP, CO, SV, SVI, and CI. ABGs: pH 7.25, $Paco_2$ 69, HCO_3^- 27, Pao_2 37. Spo_2: 64%.

A: • Pulmonary embolism and infarction (history, vital signs, hemodynamics, CXR, ECG, blood-tinged sputum, wheezing, pleural friction rub)
• Continued respiratory distress (heart rate, respiratory rate, ABGs)
• Bronchospasm (wheezing)
• Acute ventilatory failure with severe hypoxemia (ABGs)

P: Contact physician: discuss acute ventilatory failure and need for intubation and mechanical ventilation. Up-regulate oxygen therapy per protocol. Up-regulate bronchodilator therapy per protocol. Monitor and reevaluate (e.g., q30min). Remain on standby.

Discussion

Risk factors for development of a fatal pulmonary embolism include immobilization, malignant disease, and a history of thrombolic disease, including venous thrombosis, congestive heart failure, and chronic lung disease. Only about 10% of patients with pulmonary emboli do not have at least one of these risk factors. The symptoms of fatal pulmonary embolism include dyspnea (in about 60% of patients), syncope (in about 25%), altered mental status, apprehension, nonpleuritic chest pain, sweating, cough, and hemoptysis (in a smaller residue of patients).

The signs of acute pulmonary embolism include tachypnea, tachycardia, crackles, low grade temperature, lower extremity edema, hypotension, cyanosis, gallop rhythm, diaphoresis, and clinically evident phlebitis (in a progressively smaller percentage of known patients). Diagnosis of thromboembolic disease is most often made with ventilation-perfusion lung scanning, although pulmonary angiography remains the "gold standard" for diagnosis. Impedance plethysmography or duplex ultrasonography or venography of the extremities would be helpful when embolic disease is suspect from venous thrombosis in the extremities.

It is interesting to note that in surgical patients at least half the deaths due to pulmonary embolism occur within the first week after the surgical procedure, most commonly on the third to seventh day after the operation. The remainder of the deaths, however, divide equally among the second, third, and fourth postoperative weeks. The current patient certainly has one of the obvious causes for pulmonary embolism, namely, immobilization of the left leg, which was put in a cast after surgery.

At the time of the *first assessment* the patient was not in any respiratory distress. His chest physical examination was basically unremarkable, as were the chest x-ray film and arterial blood gases. The patient might well have been placed on hyperexpansion therapy, as with incentive spirometry, since his known fractures were expected to be surgically reduced. This is particularly important in the patient who is on morphine and who may be tempted to hypoventilate because of his left shoulder and left anterior chest pain and tenderness.

By the time of the *second assessment,* however, things have changed, and the patient now presents with many of the signs and symptoms listed above. The assessing therapist should recognize the seriousness of the situation from the patient's complaints, physical findings, hemodynamic parameters, and arterial blood gases. The patient's wheezing is most likely due to pulmonary embolism and infarction, as is the alveolar atelectasis. The data are abnormal enough to prompt the therapist to suggest that the patient be transferred to the ICU and to prepare for ventilator standby, since acute ventilatory failure may not be long in coming.

Indeed, in the *last assessment,* things had progressed to the point where the patient is in severe respiratory acidemia with severe hypoxemia, and mechanical ventilation becomes necessary. The treating therapist should recognize that the therapeutic options in these cases are limited by the amount of ventilation wasted in such patients because of their embolic disease. High minute ventilation may be necessary to improve (even slightly) the arterial blood gases in such patients.

Finally, it should be pointed out that wheezing due to pulmonary embolic disease is relatively rare, occurring in less than 2% of hospitalized patients. The outlook for this patient is extremely poor. Indeed, in the fifth week of this hospitalization the patient did die. The patient remained on ventilatory support up until the time of his death.

CHAPTER **15**   Flail Chest

RESPONSE 1

S: N/A (patient unconscious)

O: Vital signs: BP 165/92, HR 120, RR 26 and shallow. Paradoxical movement of the anterior chest wall. Skin: pale and cyanotic. Diminished breath sounds bilaterally. CXR: multiple double rib fractures of the right and left anterior and lateral ribs, between ribs 4 and 9; sternum fractured in three places. Atelectasis bilaterally. ABGs (nonrebreathing mask): pH 7.17, $Paco_2$ 82, HCO_3^- 27, Pao_2 37. Spo_2: 59%.

A: • Flail chest (paradoxical chest movement, CXR)
   • Atelectasis bilaterally (CXR)
   • Acute ventilatory failure with severe hypoxemia (ABGs)
   • Acute alcohol intoxication with near-fatal blood alcohol level

P: Mechanical ventilation per protocol—stat. Hyperinflation therapy per protocol. Oxygenation therapy per protocol. Monitor and reevaluate (e.g., in 1 hour).

RESPONSE 2

S: N/A

O: Cyanotic and pale. Distended neck veins. Vital signs: BP 100/65, HR 145, RR 12 (controlled). Auscultation: Right lung, absent breath sounds. Left lung, diminished breath sounds, rhonchi, and crackles. CXR: Left lung, partially aerated and patches of atelectasis. Right lung, completely atelectatic. Hemodynamics: increased CVP, RAP, $\overline{PA}$, RVSWI, and PVR and decreased PCWP, CO, SV, SVI, CI, LVSWI, and SVR. Oxygenation indices: increased $\dot{Q}s/\dot{Q}T$, $C(a-\bar{v})o_2$, and O_2ER and a decreased Do_2 and Svo_2. ABGs: pH 7.25, $Paco_2$ 65, HCO_3^- 25, Pao_2 54. Spo_2: 86%.

A: • Atelectasis: patches throughout left lung; right lung airless (CXR)
   • Increased pulmonary vascular resistance and decreased cardiac output (distended neck veins, hemodynamic indices)
   • Acute ventilatory failure with moderate hypoxemia (ABGs)
   • Poor oxygenation status (oxygenation indices)

P: Contact physician regarding patient's hemodynamic and oxygenation status; consider therapeutic bronchoscopy to treat atelectasis. Up-regulate mechanical ventilation per protocol to decrease $Paco_2$ (e.g., increase rate or volume). Up-regulate hyperinflation therapy per protocol (e.g., add positive end-expiratory pressure [PEEP]). Up-regulate oxygenation therapy per protocol. Monitor and reevaluate (e.g., in 30 to 60 minutes).

RESPONSE 3

S: N/A

O: Cyanotic and distended neck veins. Vital signs: BP 80/32, HR 190, RR 14 (controlled). Right lung: no breath sounds. Left lung: rhonchi and crackles. Large amounts of yellow sputum. ECG: premature ventricular contractions. CXR: Left lung, partially aerated with patches of atelectasis (worsening). Right lung: airless. Early signs of ARDS. Hemodynamics: worsening. ABGs: pH 7.22, $Paco_2$ 71, HCO_3^- 24, Pao_2 34. Oxygenation status: worsening. Spo_2: 61%.

A: • Atelectasis: patches throughout left lung (worsening); right lung completely atelectatic (CXR)
  • Early stages of ARDS (CXR)
  • Excessive bronchial secretions (sputum, rhonchi)
    • Infection is likely (yellow sputum)
  • Increased pulmonary vascular resistance and decreased cardiac output: worsening (distended neck veins, hemodynamic indices)
  • Acute ventilatory failure with severe hypoxemia (ABGs)
  • Poor oxygenation status: worsening (oxygenation indices)

P: Contact physician regarding patient's hemodynamic and oxygenation status; consider bronchoscopy. Up-regulate mechanical ventilation (if possible) per protocol to decrease Pa_{CO_2} (e.g., increase rate or volume). Up-regulate hyperinflation therapy per protocol. Up-regulate oxygenation therapy per protocol. Bronchial hygiene therapy per protocol. Sputum culture. Monitor and reevaluate frequently.

Discussion

This patient nicely demonstrates the sequelae of an abnormal chest wall or respiratory muscular pump. The uneven ventilation that resulted from his multiple chest fractures gave him an unstable (flail) chest, and atelectasis soon developed.

In the *first assessment* the treating therapist correctly recognizes the patient's acute ventilatory failure, intubates him, and places him on mechanical ventilation per protocol. The patient's hypoxemia is treated by increasing the ventilator oxygen concentration per protocol, and an attempt should be made to stabilize the chest still further and to treat his early atelectasis with PEEP. Many cases treated in this manner will achieve "stability" of the chest wall much sooner than one would expect, that is, within a few days. This case, however, is an exception.

The *second assessment* shows that the patient is developing signs of pulmonary hypertension with increased pulmonary vascular resistance and a low cardiac output. The right lung has become completely atelectatic despite ventilatory care. A recommendation for therapeutic bronchoscopy is certainly timely. More PEEP could be added to the ventilator settings and higher tidal volumes might well be used in such a patient. His respiratory acidosis certainly must be treated more aggressively with a change in ventilator settings.

The *third scenario* demonstrates that the patient is now slipping into ARDS and that the atelectasis noted earlier is still a problem. His blood gases have worsened despite ventilator management, and the outlook has become increasingly grim. Repeat bronchoscopic examinations are common in this setting, and it would be appropriate for the treating therapist to suggest that the procedure be repeated. If the sputum is thick, mucolytic agents may be added. Prompt culture of the sputum is an excellent idea, since the organisms may have changed while the patient has been in the hospital. Despite the aggressive care this patient received, he died 2 days later.

CHAPTER **16** Pneumothorax

RESPONSE 1

S: "I've been coughing so much and so hard my chest hurts."

O: Thin, but well nourished. Using accessory muscles of respiration. Cyanotic, digital clubbing, pursed-lip breathing, and barrel chest. Cough: frequent, strong, and productive—large amounts of thick, yellow-green sputum. Vital signs: BP 145/85, HR 94, RR 20, T 37.9° C (100.3° F). Hyperresonant percussion notes bilaterally. Diminished breath and rhonchi bilaterally. Expiration prolonged. Diminished heart sounds. PFT: moderate-to-severe obstructive pulmonary disease. CXR: translucent, flattened hemidiaphragms, and narrow heart. 10% pneumothorax between the second and third ribs on the left in the anterior axillary line. ABGs (room air): pH 7.53, $Paco_2$ 48, HCO_3^- 38, Pao_2 57 (baseline: pH 7.42, $Paco_2$ 69, HCO_3^- 41, Pao_2 74).

A:
- Exacerbation of chronic bronchitis and emphysema (history, CXR)
- Respiratory distress (vital signs, ABGs)
- Left pneumothorax: 10% (CXR)
- Excessive bronchial secretions (sputum, rhonchi)
  - Infection likely (yellow-green sputum)
- Acute alveolar hyperventilation superimposed on chronic ventilatory failure (ABGs, history)

P: Oxygenation therapy per protocol. Bronchial hygiene therapy per protocol, including sputum culture. (Specific boundaries: limited physical activity, no cough and deep breathing.) Monitor and reevaluate (e.g., in 1 hour).

RESPONSE 2

S: "I feel like hell."

O: Cyanotic, using accessory muscles of respiration, and pursed-lip breathing. Cough: frequent and weak. Patient braces himself when he coughs. Small amount of yellow-green sputum. Left anterior chest: hyperinflated and fixed. Vital signs: BP 95/55, HR 125, RR 28 and shallow. Hyperresonant notes, bilaterally. Right lung: diminished breath sounds and rhonchi; Left lung: no breath sounds. Diminished heart sounds over the right lung field. CXR: large, left-sided pneumothorax with mediastinal shift rightward. ABGs: pH 7.24, $Paco_2$ 103, HCO_3^- 43, Pao_2 37. Spo_2: 62%.

A:
- Large left-sided tension pneumothorax (CXR)
  - Treated with tube thoracotomy
- Respiratory distress (general appearance, vital signs, ABGs)
- Left lung: collapsed or atelectatic or both (CXR)
- Right lung: patches of atelectasis (CXR)
- Excessive bronchial secretions (sputum, rhonchi)
- Acute ventilatory failure superimposed on chronic ventilatory failure with severe hypoxemia (ABGs)

P: Contact physician to consider transfer to ICU. Hyperinflation therapy per protocol (e.g., CPAP mask). Oxygenation therapy per protocol. Bronchial hygiene therapy per protocol (e.g., careful nasotracheal suctioning, add acetylcysteine [Mucomyst], no chest physical therapy). Place mechanical ventilator on standby. Stay at patient's bedside. Monitor and reevaluate (e.g., in 30 minutes).

S: "I'm feeling better."

O: CXR: left lung has reexpanded about 75%; right lung has no patches of atelectasis. No longer cyanotic. Pursed-lip breathing and using accessory muscles of respiration. Right lung: rhonchi and diminished breath sounds; left lung: diminished breath sounds. Vital signs: BP 145/85, HR 105, RR 22. Hyperresonant notes bilaterally. ABGs: pH 7.35, $Paco_2$ 85, HCO_3^- 41, Pao_2 64. Spo_2: 90%.

A: • Left-sided pneumothorax: improving (CXR)
 • 25% left lung collapse or atelectasis: improving (CXR)
 • Excessive bronchial secretions (rhonchi, earlier SOAPs)
 • Chronic ventilatory failure with severe hypoxemia (ABGs)
  • ABGs not at patient's baseline level yet

P: Continue present level of hyperinflation therapy per protocol (e.g., CPAP mask). Continue present level of oxygenation therapy per protocol. Continue present level of bronchial hygiene therapy per protocol. Monitor and reevaluate (e.g., in 4-6 hours).

Discussion

The causes of pneumothorax include trauma to the chest wall, malignancy, infection of the pleural space or lung, rupture of subpleural blebs, and air leakage from tuberculous foci, or it may be without known cause (idiopathic). Pneumothoraces may be caused iatrogenically by needle tears of the pleura incurred during cutaneous needle lung biopsy or during aspiration of air or fluid from the pleural space.

This case demonstrates a pneumothorax caused by infection in a patient known to have COPD. A rupture of a subpleural bleb or leakage of air from a parenchymal lung bulla may have accounted for his problem. The patient had pneumonia 4 years ago. If the pneumonia was due to a necrotizing organism, it could have weakened the visceral pleura, allowing air leakage, although 4 years seems a bit long for that to be just showing up now.

In the *first assessment* the therapist's attention to the patient's worsening pulmonary function is appropriate. Increasing his oxygenation by use of a Venturi oxygen mask would be acceptable, as would a trial of low flow nasal cannula oxygen. The readers who recognized the small pneumothorax and noted it regarding specific boundaries for bronchial hygiene therapy are certainly worthy of positive comment. The readers who moved to get an early sputum culture knowing that prompt treatment of infection will be helpful here also deserve commendation.

Despite this, *3 hours later* the patient is clearly worsening, and indeed a stat has been called. The patient's chest x-ray film now demonstrates a left tension pneumothorax, and the therapist can help by being sure that a tube thoracostomy setup is available for the physician. The respiratory care practitioner's (RCP's) assessment comes after the chest tube has been placed and is functioning well, and he or she so records that in the assessment. The RCP notes that the compressive atelectasis noted earlier has improved and helps honor the patient's and physician's request to keep him off a ventilator if at all possible. However, the patient's CO_2 probably is high enough (103 mm Hg) to preclude this. A trial of a respiratory stimulant such as doxapram (Dopram) might be used in this setting. The therapist may try to increase the end-expiratory pressure to treat the atelectasis, but the reader should know that such therapy is fraught with the possibility of air-trapping in patients with obstructive pulmonary disease and certainly should be limited because of that.

CHAPTER **17**   Pleural Disease

S: "I cannot take a deep breath."

O: Malnourished with poor personal hygiene. Cyanotic with an occasional hacking, non-productive cough. Vital signs: BP 146/92, HR 112, RR 36 and shallow, T 37.7° C (99.8° F). Trachea slightly shifted to the left. Dull percussion notes over the right middle and right lower lung lobes. Normal vesicular breath sounds over the left lung fields and right upper lobe. No breath sounds over the right middle and right lower lobes. CXR: large, right-sided pleural effusion, right middle and right lower lobes are partially collapsed and consolidated. About 2 L of yellow fluid obtained via thoracentesis. ABGs (on 3 L/min O_2 nc): pH 7.53, $Paco_2$ 24, HCO_3^- 19, Pao_2 37. Spo_2: 64%.

A: • Right-sided pneumonia and pleural effusion (CXR)
  • Partially collapsed right middle and lower lobes, atelectasis vs. pneumonia (CXR)
• Respiratory distress (vital signs, ABGs)
• Acute alveolar hyperventilation with severe hypoxemia (ABGs)
  • Metabolic (lactic) acidosis is likely (ABGs compared to Pco_2-HCO_3^--pH relationship nomogram)

P: Hyperinflation therapy per protocol. Oxygenation therapy per protocol. Request nutrition consultation. Monitor and reevaluate.

RESPONSE 2

S: "I'm feeling better but not great yet."

O: Cyanotic and pale. Occasional dry, nonproductive cough. Vital signs: BP 135/85, HR 100, RR 24, T normal. Dull percussion notes over the right middle and right lower lobes. Normal vesicular breath sounds over the left lung and over the right upper lobe. Bronchial breath sounds over the right middle and lower lobes. CXR: small right-sided pleural effusion. Right middle and right lower lobe consolidation. ABGs: pH 7.52, $Paco_2$ 29, HCO_3^- 22, Pao_2 57. Spo_2: 89%.

A: • Small right-sided pneumonia and pleural effusion, greatly improved (CXR)
  • Atelectasis and consolidation in right middle and lower lung lobes (CXR)
• Continued respiratory distress, but improving (vital signs, ABGs)
• Acute alveolar hyperventilation with moderate hypoxemia, improved (ABGs)

P: Up-regulate hyperinflation therapy per protocol. Up-regulate oxygenation therapy per protocol. Monitor and reevaluate.

RESPONSE 3

S: "I've finally caught my breath."

O: Relaxed, alert, in semi-Fowler's position. Pale but no cyanosis. No spontaneous cough. Vital signs: 128/79, HR 88, RR 16, T normal. Dull percussion notes in right middle and right lower lung lobes. Normal vesicular breath sounds over left lung and right upper lobe. Bronchial breath sounds over right middle and right lower lobes. ABGs: pH 7.45, $Paco_2$ 36, HCO_3^- 24, Pao_2 77. Spo_2: 92%.

A: • Small right-sided pneumonia and pleural effusion, greatly improved (earlier CXR)
  • Atelectasis and consolidation in right middle and right lower lung lobes (earlier CXR)
• Normal acid-base status with mild hypoxemia (ABGs)

P: Maintain present level of hyperinflation therapy per protocol. Maintain present level of oxygenation therapy per protocol. Monitor and reevaluate (each shift).

Discussion

This case illustrates a patient with pleural effusion, one of the pleural diseases that can be helped by appropriate therapy (in this case a 2 L thoracentesis).

At the end of the *first assessment* the respiratory care practitioner still recognizes that the patient has significant respiratory morbidity. Indeed, the patient has extensive pneumonia and severe hypoxemia, despite alveolar hyperventilation. The practitioner correctly assesses the situation as one needing careful monitoring and begins oxygen therapy, presumably with a high concentration of oxygen in view of the patient's Pa_{O_2}. The practitioner recalls that the offending organism(s) is not yet identified and makes sure that sputum and thoracentesis fluid cultures are obtained.

A trial of bronchial hygiene therapy would not be incorrect, given the patient's cigarette smoking history alone or the degree of severity of the condition. In this case we admit there was no indication for such therapy in terms of the physical findings (no wheeze or expiratory prolongation). Given the patient's history, the respiratory care practitioner will also be interested in the results of the cytological studies for malignancy in both the sputum and thoracentesis fluid.

Frequently blood gases do not improve immediately after a thoracentesis, despite the fact that the fluid has been removed, because the atelectasis under the pleural effusion takes some time (hours or days) to dissipate. For this reason, hyperinflation therapy after thoracentesis is appropriate.

At the time of the *second assessment* the patient is beginning to improve, although there are signs of right middle and lower lobe consolidation. Now, good breath sounds are heard over the left lung and upper right lung, although bronchial breath sounds reflecting consolidation are still noted on the right. The respiratory therapist is now concerned that atelectasis is still present and increases the hyperinflation therapy with, perhaps, a positive expiratory pressure (PEP) mask or, possibly, with intensified incentive spirometry or intermittent positive-pressure breathing (IPPB).

In the *last assessment* the patient continues to do fairly well, although she is far from returning to baseline values. The persistent pneumonitis/atelectasis and mild hypoxemia, despite supplemental oxygen therapy, suggests the continued necessity for significant (though unchanged) therapy at this point.

This is as good a place as any to observe that often in-place therapy **does not** need to be changed at each assessment. Indeed, several series have now been reported in which appropriate therapy using the American Association for Respiratory Care (AARC) Clinical Practice Guidelines need not and should **not** be changed in about 50% to 60% of accurately performed seriatim assessments. For pedagogical reasons, we have not often taken this option in this text. However, this third assessment (in a patient with pleural effusion and underlying atelectasis/pneumonia) is a good case in point.

CHAPTER **18** Kyphoscoliosis

RESPONSE 1

S: "Trouble breathing."

O: Well nourished. Severe backward and left lateral curvature of the spine. Cyanotic, digital clubbing, and distended neck veins—especially on the right side. Cough: frequent, adequate, and productive of moderate amounts of thick, yellow sputum. Vital signs: BP 160/100, HR 90, RR 18, T 36.3° C (97.4° F). Trachea deviated to the right. Both lungs: dull percussion notes, crackles, and rhonchi. PFT: VC, FRC, and RV 45% to 50% of predicted. Hct 58%, Hb 18 g/dl. CXR: severe thoracic and spinous deformity, mediastinal shift, cor pulmonale, and bilateral infiltrates in the lung bases consistent with pneumonia and atelectasis. ABGs (room air): pH 7.52, $Paco_2$ 58, HCO_3^- 42, Pao_2 49. Spo_2: 78%.

A: • Severe kyphoscoliosis (history, CXR, ABGs, physical examination)
 • Increased work of breathing (elevated blood pressure, heart rate, and respiratory rate)
 • Excessive bronchial secretions (sputum, rhonchi)
  • Infection is likely (thick, yellow sputum)
  • Good ability to mobilize secretions (strong cough)
 • Atelectasis and consolidation (CXR)
 • Acute alveolar hyperventilation superimposed on chronic ventilatory failure with moderate hypoxemia (ABGs)
  • Possible impending ventilatory failure
 • Cor pulmonale (CXR)

P: Oxygen therapy per protocol (careful not to knock out hypoxic drive to breathe; probably should use an O_2 Venturi mask). Bronchial hygiene therapy per protocol (obtain sputum sample for culture). Contact physician regarding possible ventilatory failure. Place mechanical ventilator on standby. Monitor and reevaluate.

RESPONSE 2

S: Severe dyspnea.

O: Extreme respiratory distress. Cyanotic and perspiring. Distended neck veins. Weak, spontaneous cough. Sounds congested, but no sputum produced. Bilateral dull percussion notes, crackles, and rhonchi. Vital signs: BP 180/120, HR 130, RR 26, T 37.8° C (100° F). Hemodynamics: increased CVP, RAP, $\overline{PA}$, RVSWI, and PVR. All other hemodynamic values are normal. Oxygenation indices: increased $\dot{Q}s/\dot{Q}T$ and O_2ER and decreased Do_2 and $S\bar{v}o_2$. $\dot{V}o_2$ and $C(a-\bar{v})o_2$ are normal. ABGs: pH 7.57, $Paco_2$ 49, HCO_3^- 40, Pao_2 43. Spo_2: 76%.

A: • Severe kyphoscoliosis (history, physical exam, ABGs, CXR)
 • Increased work of breathing, worsening (increased blood pressure, heart rate, and respiratory rate)
 • Excessive bronchial secretions (rhonchi, congested cough)
 • Atelectasis and consolidation (earlier CXR)
 • Acute alveolar hyperventilation superimposed on chronic ventilatory failure with moderate-to-severe hypoxemia (ABGs and history)
  • Continued critically ill, but chances of avoiding ventilatory failure improving.

P: Up-regulate oxygen therapy per protocol (careful not to knock out hypoxic drive to breathe). Up-regulate bronchial hygiene therapy per protocol. Contact physician regarding possible ventilatory failure. Consider therapeutic bronchoscopy. Continue mechanical ventilator on standby. Monitor and reevaluate (e.g., in 1 hour)

RESPONSE 3

S: "I feel so much better. I finally have enough wind to eat some food."

O: Pale and cyanotic, but improving. Cough: strong, small amount of white sputum. Vital signs: BP 140/85, HR 83, RR 14, T normal. Crackles, rhonchi, and dull percussion notes over both lung fields; rhonchi improving. Hemodynamic and oxygenation indices improving, but still an elevated CVP, RAP, $\overline{PA}$, RVSWI, and PVR and still an increased $\dot{Q}s/\dot{Q}t$ and O_2ER and a decreased DO_2 and $S\overline{v}O_2$. CXR: improvement of the bilateral pneumonia and atelectasis. ABGs: pH 7.45, $PaCO_2$ 73, HCO_3^- 48, PaO_2 68. SpO_2: 93%.

A: • Less serious complications of severe kyphoscoliosis (history, CXR, hemodynamic and oxygenation indices, ABGs)
   • Significant improvement in problem with excessive bronchial secretions (rhonchi, cough)
   • Improvement in atelectasis and consolidation (CXR)
   • Chronic ventilatory failure with mild hypoxemia (ABGs)
     • Current ABGs likely close to patient's normal ABGs

P: Down-regulate or discontinue oxygen therapy per protocol. Down-regulate or discontinue bronchial hygiene therapy per protocol. Monitor and reevaluate (e.g., ABGs on reduced FIO_2). Recommend pulmonary rehabilitation and patient and family education (e.g., consider rocking bed, positive expiratory pressure [PEP], or cuirass respirator ventilation).

Discussion

Care of the patient with symptomatic advanced kyphoscoliosis consists of (1) treatment of the conditions that can complicate it (e.g., bronchitis, pneumonia, atelectasis, pleural effusion) and (2) treatment of the underlying condition itself.

With respect to the issue of long-term ventilatory support, the direct treatment of respiratory pump failure as it occurs in kyphoscoliotic lung disease is limited by whether the patient is willing to spend the last months or years of his or her life on a ventilator.

Initial evaluation of this patient suggests that infection is present because of the yellow sputum and recent history. The initial chest x-ray film also suggests this. Clearly respiratory failure is impending, and the therapist's desire to cautiously oxygenate the patient, give bronchial hygiene and mucolytic aerosols, and to be prepared for ventilator support are all appropriate. The patient's secondary polycythemia and cor pulmonale will improve as overall oxygenation improves, although this may take some time. The patient's hypertension may reflect CO_2 retention, which must be monitored carefully. The digital clubbing and the cor pulmonale itself suggest that the hypoxemia is of long standing.

At the time of the *second assessment* the patient still has signs of atelectasis or pneumonia despite vigorous bronchial hygiene therapy. This suggests that therapeutic bronchoscopy might be worthwhile. Although the outlook seems dismal at this point, it is the experience of many clinicians that vigorous treatment of the complicating factors (in this case hypertension and atelectasis or pneumonia) often carry the day and that the patient does recover, despite early impressions to the contrary.

This indeed seems to be the case at the time of the *last assessment*. The patient is still seen as a CO_2 retainer. Indeed the $PaCO_2$ is higher than it was on admission. However, the student should know that the high $PaCO_2$ is close to the patient's normal level. In fact, according to the pH (normal but on the alkalotic side of normal) the patient's usual $PaCO_2$ is most likely somewhat higher yet.

Comparison with baseline values would be appropriate at this time, and consideration of cuirass ventilation or a rocking bed to assist nocturnal ventilation may be in order. Ventilation could easily be assessed by oximetry at home. This case is an excellent example of the value of differentiating left-sided from right-sided cardiac failure.

CHAPTER **19** Pneumoconiosis

S: "This is the worst my breathing has ever been."

O: Vital signs: BP 182/106, HR 108, RR 32, T 38.3° C (100.8° F). Appears weak. Skin: cyanotic, damp, and clammy. Distended neck veins and digital clubbing. Cough: frequent, weak, moderate amount of thick, whitish yellow secretions. 3+ peripheral edema ankles and feet. Bilateral dull percussion notes in lung bases. Over both lungs: wheezing, rhonchi, and crackles. Pleural friction rub over the right middle lung lobe between the sixth and seventh ribs and between the anterior axillary line and midaxillary line. CXR: ground-glass appearance in the lower lobes. Calcified pleural plaques in right and left lower pleural spaces. Consolidation in right middle lung lobe. Right heart enlargement. ABGs (2 L/min O_2 nc); pH 7.56, $Paco_2$ 51, HCO_3^- 38, Pao_2 47.

A: • Respiratory distress (general appearance, vital signs, ABGs)
• Pulmonary fibrosis (history, diagnosis of asbestosis, CXR)
• Alveolar consolidation in right middle lobe (CXR, pneumonia)
• Pleurisy (asbestosis or pneumonitis) in right middle lobe (pleural friction rub)
• Excessive bronchial secretions (rhonchi, sputum production)
  • Infection likely (yellow sputum)
• Bronchospasm possible (wheezing)
  • Wheezing may be caused by bronchial secretions
• Acute alveolar hyperventilation superimposed on chronic ventilatory failure with moderate-to-severe hypoxemia (history, ABGs)
  • Possible impending ventilatory failure (ABGs).

P: Oxygen therapy per protocol. Bronchial hygiene therapy per protocol (obtain sputum culture). Trial period of bronchodilator therapy per protocol. Hyperinflation therapy per protocol. Contact physician regarding possible ventilatory failure. Monitor and reevaluate (e.g., in 1 hour).

S: N/A (patient too dyspneic to reply)

O: Condition unstable. Cough: frequent, weak, productive of thick, white and yellow secretions. Skin: cyanotic, pale, cool, and damp. Distended neck veins and peripheral edema, but improving. Vital signs: BP 192/108, HR 113, RR 34, T 38° C (100.4° F). Dull percussion notes over both lung bases. Wheezing, rhonchi, and crackles throughout both lungs. Pleural friction rub over right middle lobe between the sixth and seventh ribs and between the anterior axillary line and midaxillary line. ABGs: pH 7.57, $Paco_2$ 47, HCO_3^- 36, Pao_2 40. Spo_2: 77%.

A: • Continued respiratory distress (general appearance, vital signs, ABGs)
• Pulmonary fibrosis in lower lobes (history, diagnosis of asbestosis, recent CXR)
• Alveolar consolidation in right middle lobe (CXR, pneumonia)
• Pleurisy or pneumonia that has extended into pleural space over right middle lobe (pleural friction rub)
• Excessive bronchial secretions (rhonchi, sputum production)
  • Infection likely (yellow sputum)
• Bronchospasm possible (wheezing)
  • Wheezing not improving in response to bronchodilator treatment
  • Wheezing may be caused by bronchial secretions
• Acute alveolar hyperventilation superimposed on chronic ventilatory failure with severe hypoxemia, worsening (history, ABGs)
  • Possible impending ventilatory failure (ABGs)

P: Up-regulate oxygen therapy per protocol. Up-regulate bronchial hygiene therapy per protocol. Continue trial period of bronchodilator therapy per protocol. Continue or increase frequency of hyperinflation therapy per protocol. Monitor and reevaluate (e.g., repeat ABGs in 30 minutes).

RESPONSE 3

S: N/A (intubated on ventilator)

O: Vital signs: BP 135/90, HR 84, T 38.3° C (100.8° F). Frequent premature ventricular contractions. Skin: pale, cyanotic, and clammy. Distended neck veins. Peripheral edema: ankles and feet. Dull percussion notes over the lung bases. Wheezing, rhonchi, and crackles throughout both lungs. Thick, greenish yellow sputum frequently suctioned. Pleural friction rub over the right middle lung lobe between the sixth and seventh ribs and between the anterior axillary line and midaxillary line. Hemodynamics: elevated CVP, RAP, $\overline{PA}$, RVSWI, and PVR. ABGs: pH 7.53, Pa_{CO_2} 56, HCO_3^- 38, Pa_{O_2} 246. Sp_{O_2}: 98%.

A:
- Pulmonary fibrosis, lower lung lobes (history, diagnosis of asbestosis, recent CXR)
- Alveolar consolidation, right middle lobe (recent CXR showing pneumonia)
- Pneumonia has possibly extended into pleural space over right middle lobe (pleural friction rub)
- Excessive bronchial secretions (rhonchi, sputum production)
  - Infection likely (greenish yellow sputum, possibly new organism)
  - Bronchospasm possible (wheezing)
  - Wheezing not improving in response to bronchodilator treatment
  - Wheezing may be caused by bronchial secretions
- Acute alveolar hyperventilation superimposed on chronic ventilatory failure and overly corrected hypoxemia (ABGs)
  - Excessive mechanical ventilation and oxygenation

P: Down-regulate oxygenation therapy per protocol (e.g., decrease F_{IO_2}). Down-regulate mechanical ventilation (e.g., decrease rate or tidal volume). Continue bronchial hygiene therapy per protocol (sputum culture). Continue trial period of bronchodilator therapy per protocol. Continue or up-regulate hyperinflation therapy per protocol (depending on mean airway pressure). Monitor and reevaluate (e.g., in 30 minutes).

Discussion

The admitting history reveals that the patient has been diagnosed with moderate pneumoconiosis (probable asbestosis) and that he has been a heavy smoker for more than 40 years. It is no surprise that the pulmonary function tests in the past have shown mild-to-moderate obstructive and restrictive pulmonary disorders.

What is new is the history of congestive heart failure and the arterial blood gases on his discharge from the hospital 10 months before this admission, which demonstrated chronic ventilatory failure. The patient's recent fever and cough before his emergency room admission suggest an infectious cause for his symptoms. His cyanosis, neck vein distension, and digital clubbing suggest chronic hypoxemia. The sputum secretions confirm that infection may indeed be present and that the assessing therapist's desire to obtain a sputum culture is appropriate. The pleural rub demonstrated by this patient could be related to his asbestosis or to pneumonic infiltrate extending to the pleural surface.

In the *initial assessment* the patient's severe hypertension and his fever should have been noted. Both deserve vigorous therapy if his pulmonary function is to improve at all. The patient is hyperventilating with respect to his earlier outpatient blood gases. This assessment should record the patient's underlying pulmonary conditions (chronic pulmonary fibrosis, bronchitis, and congestive heart failure) but should really zero in on the treatable issues, specifically the pulmonary infection as suggested by the sputum and chest x-ray film.

At the time of the *second evaluation* the patient's hypoxemia has worsened despite oxygen therapy. If not already being used, Venturi oxygen mask therapy would be indicated here, and additional mucolytics and endobronchial suctioning may also be indicated. The trial of hyperinflation therapy would have to be made carefully, given the patient's known airway obstruction. A trial of diuretic therapy to reduce the cor pulmonale may have been ordered by the physician. The therapist's opinion that the wheezing might be caused by bronchial secretions, rather than by out-and-out bronchospasm, very possibly is correct. However, the distinction is academic, as both bronchodilator therapy and mucolytics might be used in this setting.

The *last assessment* reveals that the patient has slipped into acute ventilatory failure with near cardiopulmonary arrest and ventricular arrhythmias. The patient is then intubated and taken to the ICU, where more aggressive cardiovascular monitoring and ventilatory care can be delivered. Note that at the time of this evaluation the patient's chest x-ray film has not yet been reviewed or interpreted. Because of the patient's precarious condition the therapist should take it on himself or herself to request that this be done promptly.

The change in the patient's sputum color from thick and white to greenish yellow suggests superinfection with another organism, and reculture of the sputum is appropriate. The patient is hyperoxygenated, and the F_{IO_2} should be reduced appropriately. Ventilator parameters should be adjusted to provide good pulmonary expansion while avoiding high mean airway pressures. Despite all that could be done for this patient, he died as a result of left congestive heart failure and pneumonia complicating his pulmonary asbestosis.

CHAPTER **20** Cancer of the Lungs

S: "I've coughed up a cup of sputum since breakfast."

O: Vital signs: BP 155/85, HR 90, RR 22, T normal. Perspiring and appears weak and cyanotic. Voice sounds hoarse. Weak cough. Large amounts of blood-streaked sputum. Dull percussion notes over the left lower lobe. Rhonchi, wheezing, and crackles throughout both lung fields. Recent PFT: restrictive and obstructive pulmonary disorder. CT scan and CXR: 2 to 5 cm masses in right and left mediastinum in hilar regions and atelectasis of left lower lobe. Bronchoscopy: protruding tumors in both left and right large airways, mucus plugging. Biopsy: squamous cell bronchogenic carcinoma. ABGs (2 L/min O_2 nc) pH 7.51, $Paco_2$ 29, HCO_3^- 22, Pao_2 66. Spo_2: 92%.

A: • Bronchogenic carcinoma (CT scan and biopsy)
• Respiratory distress (vital signs, ABGs)
• Excessive bloody bronchial secretions (sputum, rhonchi)
  • Mucus plugging likely (bronchoscopy)
• Poor ability to mobilize secretions (weak cough)
• Atelectasis of left lower lobe (CXR)
• Acute alveolar hyperventilation with mild hypoxemia (ABGs)

P: Oxygenation therapy per protocol. Hyperinflation therapy per protocol. Bronchial hygiene therapy per protocol. Monitor and reevaluate soon and regularly (e.g., in 1 to 2 hours).

S: "I'm still not breathing very well."

O: Vital signs: BP 166/90, HR 95, RR 28, T normal. Vomiting over past 10 hours. Cyanotic, tired, and damp from perspiration. Cough: weak and productive of moderately thick, clear and white sputum. Dull percussion notes over both the right and left lower lobes. Rhonchi, wheezing, and crackles over both lung fields. ABGs: pH 7.55, $Paco_2$ 25, HCO_3^- 20, Pao_2 53. Spo_2: 88%.

A: • Bronchogenic carcinoma (earlier CT scan and biopsy)
• Not tolerating chemotherapy well (excessive vomiting)
• Continued respiratory distress
• Excessive bronchial secretions (sputum, rhonchi)
  • Mucus plugging still likely (earlier bronchoscopy, secretions becoming thicker)
• Poor ability to mobilize secretions (weak cough)
• Atelectasis of left lower lobes. Atelectasis likely in right lower lobe now (CXR, dull percussion notes)
• Acute alveolar hyperventilation with moderate hypoxemia, worsening (ABGs)
  • Possible ventilatory failure

P: Up-regulate oxygenation therapy per protocol. Up-regulate hyperinflation therapy per protocol. Up-regulate bronchial hygiene therapy per protocol. Contact physician about possible ventilatory failure. Consider therapeutic bronchoscopy. Monitor and reevaluate.

RESPONSE 3

S: N/A (patient comatose)

O: Unresponsive. Pale, cyanotic, and perspiring. No cough noted. Rhonchi heard without stethoscope. Vital signs: BP 170/105, HR 110, RR 11 and shallow, T normal. Rhonchi, wheezing, and crackles over both lung fields. ABGs: pH 7.28, $Paco_2$ 63, HCO_3^- 27, Pao_2 66. Spo_2: 90%.

A:
- Bronchogenic carcinoma (earlier CT scan and biopsy)
- Excessive bronchial secretions (rhonchi)
  - Mucus plugging still likely (earlier bronchoscopy, rhonchi)
- Poor ability to mobilize secretions (no cough)
- Atelectasis (history)
- Acute ventilatory failure with mild hypoxemia (ABGs)

P: Contact physician about acute ventilatory failure (discuss code status). Up-regulate oxygenation therapy per protocol. Up-regulate hyperinflation therapy per protocol. Up-regulate bronchial hygiene therapy per protocol. May choose not to be aggressive at this time. Monitor and reevaluate.

Discussion

This case demonstrates the few specific treatments that a respiratory care practitioner can bring to his care of patients with lung cancer. Specifically, it illustrates that most of the patients have concomitant obstructive pulmonary disease with need for good bronchial hygiene therapy. The patient's comfort must be kept in mind at all times.

The *first assessment* is performed soon after bronchoscopy, and a diagnosis had been made. The patient's blood-stained sputum may reflect the primary tumor or, more likely, bleeding from the bronchoscopy sites. The practitioner will need to watch this as the day goes along. No improvement in the patient's wheezing can be expected if endobronchial tumor is the cause, but it may improve if the obstructive pulmonary disease (from cigarette smoking) is the causative factor.

The rhonchi, wheezing, and crackles indicate the need for vigorous bronchial hygiene therapy. The atelectasis in the left lower lobe suggests that a trial of careful hyperinflation therapy is in order. The ABGs drawn on 2 L/min O_2 show moderate hypoxemia, despite alveolar hyperventilation. A trial of oxygen by Venturi mask (or nonrebreathing mask) would be helpful. The patient's anxiety may be alleviated with appropriate treatment of the hypoxemia.

The *second assessment* reveals that the patient may now have atelectasis in both the right and left lower lobes (recall where the tumor masses were noted earlier). This may be a setting in which therapeutic bronchoscopy or laser-assisted endobronchial resection of the tumor masses may be helpful. The patient continues to be hypoxemic, despite alveolar hyperventilation. A higher Fio_2 (through a Venturi oxygen mask) may be indicated. Vigorous suctioning should be done. It would not be surprising if at least one cycle of ventilator support would be ordered for such a patient, given the fact that the patient has just received radiation and chemotherapy. His wishes in this respect should be checked against his living will or durable power of attorney for health care if such a document exists.

The *last assessment* indicates that the patient did not elect this type of therapy and that he is now slipping into acute ventilatory failure. All have agreed that the patient is close to death. The practitioner may be excused for not suggesting the use of pulmonary percussion at this time given the patient's wishes. If, however, aggressive therapy was still in order, formal evaluation and treatment of superimposed atelectasis or pneumonia or both would be in order.

CHAPTER 21   Adult Respiratory Distress Syndrome

S: Complains of moderate dyspnea.

O: Vital signs: BP 125/78, HR 93, RR 21, T normal. Skin: pale. No cough. Nonproductive voluntary cough. Tenderness over anterior chest. Bilateral lung fields: dull percussion notes, bronchial breath sounds. Spo_2: 95%. ABGs (3 L/min O_2 nc): pH 7.51, $Paco_2$ 29, HCO_3^- 22, Pao_2 68. CXR: bilateral "ground glass" infiltrates worsening.

A: • Increased work of breathing (vital signs, ABGs)
   • Increased lung infiltrates: possible atelectasis or consolidation? Possible ARDS? Fat emboli? (CXR, chest assessment findings)
   • Acute alveolar hyperventilation with mild hypoxemia (ABGs)

P: Hyperinflation therapy per protocol. Oxygen therapy per protocol. Monitor and reevaluate (e.g., in 30 to 60 minutes with ABGs)

S: "I'm feeling worse."

O: Vital signs: RR 30, BP 165/90, HR 110, T 38.8° C (101.8° F). Tender anterior chest. Bronchial breath sounds and crackles bilaterally. Spo_2: 75%. ABGs: pH 7.56, $Paco_2$ 24, HCO_3^- 18, and Pao_2 35.

A: • Continued increased work of breathing (vital signs, ABGs)
   • Worsening of atelectasis or pneumonia (chest assessment, bronchial breath sounds and crackles)
   • Acute alveolar hyperventilation with moderate hypoxemia (ABGs)
     • Impending acute ventilatory failure (ABGs)

P: Contact physician regarding impending ventilatory failure. Up-regulate hyperinflation therapy per protocol (if tolerated). Up-regulate oxygen therapy per protocol. Review chest x-ray film just taken. Monitor and reevaluate (e.g., in 1 hour).

S: N/A (patient unarousable)

O: Vital signs: RR 18, BP 170/97, HR 150, T 37.8° C (100° F). Skin: cyanotic. No verbal response. Bronchial breath sounds and crackles bilaterally. Spo_2: 69%. ABGs: pH 7.31, $Paco_2$ 48, HCO_3^- 22, Pao_2 31. CXR: Increased infiltrates bilaterally.

A: • Worsening of interstitial lung process: ARDS or atelectasis vs. pneumonia (chest assessment, CXR)
   • Acute ventilatory failure with moderate hypoxemia (ABGs)

P: Contact physician. Prepare for immediate intubation and mechanical ventilation. Continue hyperinflation therapy per mechanical ventilator protocol. Intensify oxygen therapy per protocol. Monitor and reevaluate closely.

Discussion

Multiple trauma (including chest wall trauma) in a patient should in itself constitute notification to the therapist that his expertise will be needed. In this patient, who is hypotensive and has fractured teeth along with multiple bone fractures, three diagnoses should immediately come to mind: (1) the patient's potential for developing adult respiratory distress syndrome (ARDS), (2) the possibility that dental fragments were aspirated, causing obstructive pneumonia or atelectasis, and (3) fat emboli, which could well complicate an already serious situation.

At the time of the *first evaluation* the development of progressive hypoxemia, "ground glass" infiltrates in the chest film, and increasing dyspnea 24 hours or so after multiple trauma are almost pathognomonic of ARDS. Examination and assessment have determined that despite his frontal chest injury, the patient does *not* have a flail chest. The probability that the patient will require intubation and mechanical ventilation with positive end-expiratory pressure (PEEP) or inverse ratio ventilation is high.

A trial of hyperinflation therapy (e.g., with mask continuous positive airway pressure [CPAP]) is indicated in this setting but is often not successful because of patient intolerance. Preparation should be made for intubation and mechanical ventilation in the event there is any further decrease in the pulmonary function. Initially the patient should be placed on mask oxygen therapy to improve oxygenation and to supply him with a known F_{IO_2}, so that the alveolar-arterial oxygen gradient can be calculated (knowing that the patient will likely be refractory, to some degree, to oxygen therapy). Hyperinflation therapy with incentive spirometry or intermittent positive-pressure breathing (IPPB) is indicated but probably would not be well tolerated because of chest pain. Prompt (30 to 60 minutes) reevaluation with repeat ABGs is indicated.

At the time of the *second evaluation* 3 days after surgery, the patient has not improved and, indeed, is feeling worse. He is cyanotic and tachypneic, and his arterial blood gases show profound deterioration, with a Pa_{O_2} of 35 mm Hg and a Pa_{CO_2} of 24 mm Hg. An attempt may now be made to increase his hyperinflation therapy with a positive expiratory pressure (PEP) mask or CPAP, but it will probably be futile. If the patient is not on an F_{IO_2} of 1.0, he should be. Review of the chest film is mandatory, since a complicating problem such as a pneumothorax could, theoretically, have occurred, or a large pleural effusion could have developed. If the reader is ready to intubate the patient at this point, it is justified.

The *last evaluation* occurs 30 minutes after the second one. The patient is now unresponsive. His auscultatory findings have not changed, but his blood gases have deteriorated still further. If protocol allows, the patient should be immediately intubated. If not, the attending physician should be called to request intubation and the immediate start of mechanical ventilation.

With this aggressive therapy the patient gradually improved. He remained on a mechanical ventilator for 14 days and then spent an additional 1 month recovering in the hospital. During this recovery another pulmonary insult in the form of an acute pulmonary embolus developed. He was eventually discharged home on supplemental oxygen and was subsequently lost to follow-up.

◆◆ KEY POINT ANSWERS   **For ARDS (DRG 99/100)**

1. Basic Concept Formation

a. *Trauma* is associated with flail chest, pulmonary contusion, pulmonary emboli, pneumothorax, and ARDS.

b. *Infection* is associated with pneumonia, empyema, and ARDS.

c. *Yes.*

2. Data Base Formation

a. First described clearly in 1967, ARDS has been associated with the following conditions:

   (1) Sepsis or sepsis syndrome (systemic inflammatory response syndrome [SIRS])
   (2) Gastric aspiration
   (3) Trauma
   (4) Heroin and other drug overdose
   (5) Multiple transfusions
   (6) Fat emboli
   (7) Chemical or smoke inhalation
   (8) Burns
   (9) Disseminated intravascular coagulation (DIC)
   (10) Viral pneumonia
   (11) Pancreatitis
   (12) Drug reactions
   (13) Near drowning

b. *SIRS* has recently been identified by the presence of two or more of the following criteria:

   (1) Body *temperature* >38° C (100.4° F) or <36° C (98.6° F)
   (2) *Heart rate* > 90 beats per minute
   (3) *Tachypnea:* respiratory rate >20 breaths per minute or $Paco_2$ <32 mm Hg.
   (4) Alterations in white blood cell count (WBC): >12,000/mm^3 or <4,000/mm^3 or the presence of >10% immature neutrophils (bands).

   SIRS is an evolving process, involving multiple organ failure (MOF) at sites remote from the initial insult. ARDS is but one expression of SIRS/MOF.

c. ARDS produces acute *inflammation of the alveolar-capillary membrane** with *hyaline membrane formation, atelectasis,* and an element of *alveolar consolidation. Pulmonary hypertension and right-sided heart failure* may also occur.

d. Following injury to the pulmonary capillary endothelium or the alveolar epithelium, *high pormeability pulmonary edema* (HPPE) occurs. (1) The chest x-ray film reveals diffuse, bilateral "ground glass" infiltrates, (2) extravascular water increases, and (3) *static lung compliance falls.* The pulmonary capillary end-diastolic ("wedge") pressures are normal. *Severe, oxygen-resistant hypoxemia* (shunt physiology) develops.

e. The goals of therapy are to *treat hypoxemia, stabilize alveolar size, and treat respiratory failure.*

f. Treatment of ARDS is supportive and consists of *oxygen therapy, mechanical ventilation, and PEEP.* The use of *aerosolized surfactant* is undergoing evaluation. This substance is reduced in ARDS, as it is in the neonatal respiratory distress syndrome (IRDS/NRDS).

g. Following are the expected outcomes, possible adverse effects, and monitors of protocols you selected:

Protocol	Expected Outcomes	Possible Adverse Effects	Monitors
Oxygen Therapy (see box, p. 6)	Improved hypoxemia	Pulmonary oxygen toxicity	ECG, Spo_2, ABGs
PEEP	Improved static compliance, hypoxemia	Barotrauma	Spo_2, static compliance, ABGs
Mechanical ventilation	Improved Pao_2, $Paco_2$	Barotrauma	ECG, Spo_2, static compliance, ABGs

3. Assessment

a. *Yes.* He had modest tachycardia and tachypnea, bilateral "ground glass" pulmonary infiltrates, and definite hypoxemia on 3 L/min oxygen, despite alveolar hyperventilation. What was earlier thought to be a pulmonary contusion had clearly now progressed.

---

*See color plate 22 in Des Jardins T, Burton GG: *Clinical manifestations and assessment of respiratory disease,* ed 3, St Louis, 1995, Mosby.

b. *Yes.* There was extensive trauma to multiple bones and organs, and surgery was prolonged.

c. *Yes.* He demonstrated the effects of *relative shunt physiology, reduced lung compliance, and alveolar inflammation,* which should all have been clear by the time of the *second assessment.*

d. ARDS is a *severe disease* by definition.

e. Pulmonary *infectious complications* account for most ARDS deaths. During the course of the illness presented in these three scenarios, this patient had not yet developed them. He eventually did develop *pulmonary embolic disease,* which is a known complication of trauma and prolonged immobilization. He never did develop *chronic ventilatory failure,* which is seen in a small number of ARDS patients.

4. **Application**

   a. Oxygen therapy **was** indicated from the start because of the patient's *hypoxemia.*

   b. Monitoring **was** indicated because of the patient's *hypoxemia and overall status.*

   c. Hyperinflation therapy **was** indicated to *stabilize the atelectasis-prone alveoli.*

5. **Evaluation**

   a. Following are the expected results of each aspect of therapy selected:

      (1) *Satisfactory oxygenation* (Sa_{O_2}, 90%) should result from use of the Oxygen Therapy Protocol.

      (2) *Adequate gas exchange* should occur when you institute mechanical ventilation or PEEP. An attempt should be made to keep mean airway pressures as low as possible; *permissive hypercapnia* may be necessary.

   b. See *Monitors* listed in Answer 2.g.

   c. *Oxygen therapy* as listed can be carried up to an $F_{I_{O_2}}$ of 1.0. *Mask CPAP* can be tried in the short term but is generally poorly tolerated because of aerophagia and pressure discomfort from the mask. Unfortunately, mechanical ventilation or PEEP therapy, with its attendant costs and hazards, is almost always necessary in these patients.

   d. The risks of mechanical ventilation therapy are *barotrauma* and *oxygen toxicity* from prolonged high-concentration oxygen therapy.

   e. If the patient improves, the ventilator $F_{I_{O_2}}$ is reduced first; then the PEEP is tapered; then pressure support ventilation (PSV) weaning is started.

   f. If the patient does not improve on high PEEP, or high $F_{I_{O_2}}$ therapy, specialized centers may try extracorporeal membrane oxygenation *(ECMO)* or *nitrous oxide ventilation.*

6. **Boundary Awareness**

   a. *Increasing pulmonary infiltrates* on chest x-ray films, a *widening alveolar-arterial oxygen gradient,* and *falling static pulmonary compliance are signs of worsening* in ARDS.

   b. Probably at the time of the *first assessment,* as these patients progress downhill rapidly in the early stages of ARDS.

   c. Certainly by the time of the *second assessment,* when it is clear that the patient has ARDS.

   d. *Serial ABG determinations* document acute ventilatory failure, which was seen at the time of the *third assessment.*

   e. *Barotrauma, secondary pulmonary infection, and oxygen toxicity* are all risks of therapy and are not uncommon.

CHAPTER 22 Idiopathic (infant) Respiratory Distress Syndrome

RESPONSE 1

S: NA

O: Mild respiratory distress: intercostal retractions, nasal flaring, and cyanosis. Vital signs: RR 74, BP 50/20, HR 180. Grunting breath sounds and crackles bilaterally. CXR: mild haziness in lung bases. ABGs (F_{IO_2} 0.4): pH 7.52, Pa_{CO_2} 29, HCO_3^- 21, Pa_{O_2} 49.

A: • Impending infant respiratory distress syndrome (history, CXR).
• Atelectasis, consolidation, and hyaline membrane formation likely (history, CXR).
• Acute alveolar hyperventilation with moderate-to-severe hypoxemia (ABGs).

P: Hyperinflation therapy per protocol. Oxygenation therapy per protocol. Administration of exogenous surfactant per protocol. Monitor (e.g., vital signs, breath sounds, and acute changes in color and muscle tone) and evaluate closely. Place infant ventilator on standby.

RESPONSE 2

S: NA

O: Vital signs: RR 30 (ventilator), BP 60/40, HR 184. Harsh, bronchial breath sounds and fine crackles bilaterally. CXR: dense, ground-glass appearance in both lungs. ABGs (F_{IO_2} 0.6): pH 7.28, Pa_{CO_2} 53, HCO_3^- 19, Pa_{O_2} 57.

A: • Infant respiratory distress syndrome (history, CXR).
• Worsening of atelectasis, consolidation, and hyaline membrane formation likely (history, CXR).
• Acute ventilatory failure with severe hypoxemia (ABGs).

P: Continue hyperinflation therapy per protocol. Up-regulate oxygenation therapy per protocol. Continue the administration of exogenous surfactant per protocol. Constantly monitor ventilator settings to correct acute ventilatory failure (e.g., increase rate or tidal volume). Monitor and reevaluate closely.

RESPONSE 3

S: NA

O: Vital signs: RR 42, BP 74/50, HR 120. Normal vesicular breath sounds. CXR: normal. ABGs: pH 7.42, Pa_{CO_2} 37, HCO_3^- 24, Pa_{O_2} 162.

A: • It appears that atelectasis, consolidation, and hyaline membrane are no longer present (history, CXR).
• Normal ventilatory status with overoxygenation (ABGs).

P: Down-regulate hyperinflation therapy per protocol. Down-regulate oxygen therapy per protocol. Monitor and reevaluate.

Discussion

IRDS is one of the most common complications of prematurity. It can be avoided with aggressive respiratory care. IRDS is often referred to as *hyaline membrane disease* because of the formation of a hyaline membrane inside the alveoli. The problem is also complicated by inadequate surfactant production. The low levels of surfactant in the presence of immature lung tissue produce atelectasis. Hypoxia and pulmonary hypertension develop, which keeps the ductus arteriosus patent and thus allows continuation of fetal circulation after birth. The low Apgar scores upon delivery are also an indication of impending respiratory distress. At this point, hypercapnia and respiratory acidosis occur, which ultimately may be fatal.

IRDS often is due to lack of prenatal care for the mother. In this case the premature delivery could have been stopped medically with tocolytic drugs such as terbutaline. The fact that the mother smoked throughout the pregnancy decreased the level of oxygen available to the infant, possibly resulting in the infant's being small for gestational age. The mother's youth in this case is also an indication that there may be a high incidence of complications with the birth.

Initially the low Apgar score indicates that the infant needs constant monitoring. Although cyanosis and crackles are normal signs immediately following delivery, the nasal flaring and intercostal retractions are not. These signs, along with the grunting respirations, are an indication of impending respiratory failure. The blood pressure is normal, but the infant shows signs of tachypnea and tachycardia, which indicate increased work of breathing. The infant will need an intravenous infusion started stat, as dehydration and humidification will be additional problems. The infant should also be placed in an open-bed radiant warmer so that a neutral thermal environment is provided immediately.

At the 16-hour assessment the infant is placed on mechanical ventilation because of the clinical findings. Since another dose of surfactant has probably been administered to the child, nasal CPAP could be tried before intubation and placement on the ventilator. Nasal CPAP does not require the passing of a tube through the vocal cords yet aids in the distribution of the surfactant into the distal alveoli.

The last assessment shows that the treatment has worked and that the infant continues to improve. The vital signs are all within the normal range; the ABGs indicate that the F_{IO_2} can continue to be decreased; and the infant can successfully be weaned from mechanical ventilation. The only concern (at this point) is the high Pa_{O_2}, since a value less than 100 mm Hg is required to avoid retinopathy of prematurity.

The use of surfactant and the PEEP or CPAP pressures for aerosol distribution successfully reversed the infant's condition. The short time needed to reverse the IRDS will preclude any permanent damage to the lungs, which might have occurred if the infant had remained on the ventilator and developed bronchopulmonary dysplasia.

CHAPTER 23 Chronic Interstitial Lung Disease

RESPONSE 1

S: "I had to stop taking my aerobic class because of shortness of breath."

O: Vital signs: BP 145/90, HR 96, RR 28, T normal. Cyanotic, digital clubbing. Frequent, dry, nonproductive cough. Peripheral edema, distended neck veins, and enlarged and tender liver. Pursed-lip breathing. Bilateral bronchial breath sounds and crackles. Tactile and vocal fremitus over lung bases. PFTs: moderate restrictive and obstructive disorder; 50% reduction in D_{LCO}. CXR: bilateral diffuse interstitial infiltrates and nodular densities in lower lung lobes, air bronchograms, right ventricular cardiomegaly. ABGs (room air): pH 7.53, $Paco_2$ 29, HCO_3^- 21, Pao_2 61.

A: • Moderate respiratory distress (history, vital signs, ABGs)
• Bilateral interstitial infiltrates (CXR)
• Bronchial obstruction, possibly bronchospasm (PFT)
• Cor pulmonale (CXR)
• Acute alveolar hyperventilation with mild-to-moderate hypoxemia (ABGs)

P: Oxygen therapy per protocol. Trial period of hyperinflation therapy per protocol. Trial of bronchodilator therapy per protocol. Monitor and reevaluate (e.g., per shift)

RESPONSE 2

S: "I want to leave the hospital."

O: Appears weak and tired. Cough: frequent, dry. Pursed-lip breathing and cyanotic nail beds. Vital signs: BP 142/91, HR 90, RR 23, T normal. Bilateral bronchial breath sounds and crackles. PEFR: 280 before and after bronchodilator therapy. CXR: bilateral diffuse interstitial infiltrates and nodular densities in lower lung lobes and air bronchograms. Right ventricular cardiomegaly. Histology report: sarcoidosis. Gallium scan positive. ABGs: pH 7.48, $Paco_2$ 32, HCO_3^- 23, Pao_2 67. Spo_2: 94%.

A: • Moderate respiratory distress (general observation, vital signs, ABGs)
• Bilateral interstitial infiltrates (CXR)
• Active sarcoidosis (histology report, CXR, gallium scan)
• Bronchial obstruction (PEFR), probably from sarcoidosis
• Acute alveolar hyperventilation with mild hypoxemia (ABGs)

P: Up-regulate oxygenation therapy per protocol. Discontinue hyperinflation and bronchodilator therapy per protocol (with the confirmation of sarcoidosis, the effectiveness of hyperinflation and bronchodilator therapy is questionable). Continue to monitor and reevaluate (e.g., each shift)

RESPONSE 3

S: "I feel much better."

O: No longer in respiratory distress (on present O_2 setting). Cough: frequent, dry, and hacking. Pursed-lip breathing and cyanosis. Vital signs: BP 133/86, HR 86, RR 15, T normal. Bronchial breath sounds bilaterally. CXR: bilateral diffuse interstitial infiltrates and nodular densities; air bronchograms were also seen. ABGs: pH 7.44, $Paco_2$ 36, HCO_3^- 23, Pao_2 84. Spo_2: 95%.

A: • Bilateral interstitial infiltrates (CXR)
      • Sarcoidosis (histology report)
      • Bronchial obstruction (PEFR)
      • Normal acid-base status with corrected hypoxemia (ABGs)

P: Recommend home care oxygenation therapy per protocol. Schedule exercise oxygen titration study. Check pneumococcal and influenza vaccine status.

Discussion

Respiratory care of the patient with chronic interstitial lung disease involves ensuring adequate oxygenation, reversing or preventing atelectasis, and treating any obstructive component that may be present. Two interstitial lung diseases have a strong obstructive component: sarcoidosis and cystic fibrosis (see Chapter 6).

The *first assessment* suggests that hypoxemia and cor pulmonale may be complicating the patient's course early in the disease. Thus oxygen therapy is certainly indicated. While the workup is proceeding, not much more can be done to treat her illness. This patient was undiagnosed when she came to the clinic, and it would be some time before the effects of corticosteroid therapy would be felt.

In the *second assessment* a gallium scan indicates that the patient has cytoactive sarcoidosis, for which corticosteroid therapy might be helpful. The patient is modestly hypoxic, and oxygen therapy should be up-regulated. There has been no improvement in wheezing or crackles. Thus hyperinflation and bronchodilator therapy can safely be discontinued. These were instituted only on a trial basis.

At the time of the *third assessment,* with continued improvement in oxygenation with appropriate oxygen therapy, all that remains is to prepare for discharge of this patient on a simple program of supplemental oxygen therapy if indicated. An oxygen titration study is appropriate for this purpose. This patient should now be recognized as having chronic lung disease, no matter what her symptom status. This patient is now at the age where both pneumococcal vaccine and influenza vaccine should be given. The pneumococcal vaccine can be given at any time of the year and should be repeated every 5 to 10 years in patients with a chronic lung disease. Influenza vaccine should be given yearly during the fall months. A note should be added to the patient's chart that this has been recommended.

The fact that this patient presented with cor pulmonale suggests that a significant amount of parenchymal lung damage already exists and that supplemental oxygen therapy may be needed for a long time, if not for the remainder of the patient's lifetime.

CHAPTER **24** Guillain-Barré Syndrome

S: NA (intubated on the ventilator)

O: Vital signs: BP 126/82, HR 68. No spontaneous breaths. CXR: normal. Normal breath sounds. ABGs: pH 7.51, $Paco_2$ 29, HCO_3^- 22, Pao_2 204. Spo_2: 98%.

A: • Acute alveolar hyperventilation with excessive oxygenation (ABGs)
  • Inappropriate ventilator settings
    • Excessive alveolar ventilation (increased pH and decreased $Paco_2$)
    • Fio_2 too high (ABGs)

P: Adjust mechanical ventilator setting (e.g., decrease tidal volume and Fio_2) according to protocol. Monitor closely and reevaluate.

S: N/A

O: Skin color good. Crackles and rhonchi over both lung fields. Moderate amount of white, clear secretions being suctioned on a regular basis. Vital signs: BP 124/83, HR 74, T 37.7° C (99.8° F). CXR: unremarkable. ABGs: pH 7.44, $Paco_2$ 35, HCO_3^- 24, and Pao_2 98. Spo_2: 97%.

A: • Normal acid-base and oxygenation status on present ventilator settings (ABGs)
  • Excessive sputum accumulation; may progress to mucus plugging and atelectasis (crackles, rhonchi, white and clear secretions)

P: Begin bronchial hygiene therapy per protocol (sputum stain and culture). Hyperinflation therapy per protocol (to offset any early development of atelectasis). Monitor and reevaluate (e.g., per shift).

S: N/A

O: Skin color good. Crackles and rhonchi over both lung fields improving. Small amount of clear secretions suctioned. Vital signs: BP 118/79, HR 68, T normal. No spontaneous respirations. CXR: normal. ABGs: pH 7.42, $Paco_2$ 37, HCO_3^- 24, Pao_2 97. Spo_2: 97%.

A: • Normal acid-base and oxygenation status on present ventilator settings (ABGs)
  • Respiratory muscle pump insufficiency (no spontaneous respirations)
  • Sputum accumulation improving (crackles, rhonchi, clear secretions)

P: Continue bronchial hygiene therapy per protocol. Continue hyperinflation therapy per protocol. Monitor and reevaluate (e.g., forced vital capacity [FVC], forced expiratory volume in 1 second [FEV_1], negative inspiratory force [NIF] per shift)

Discussion

Guillain-Barré syndrome is a neuromuscular paralysis that ensues after infection from a neurotropic virus. This patient has a classic history of ascending paralysis and paresthesias and the diagnostic finding of albuminocytologic dissociation in the spinal fluid. In this setting, serial FVC maneuvers must be charted. Once respiratory failure supervenes, intubation and respiratory support on a ventilator become necessary.

By the time of the *first assessment,* early CO_2 retention was present, and given the clinical setting, the patient was appropriately intubated. The initial blood gases show hyperoxia and hyperventilation. An appropriate response would be to adjust the ventilator settings by reducing the tidal volume or frequency or both and the F_{IO_2}. At the time of this assessment the patient exhibited no evidence of airways obstruction or secretions. Therefore bronchial hygiene therapy was not indicated. Indeed, all that needed to be done was to assure adequate ventilation and oxygenation on the ventilator.

However, 3 days later, at the time of the *second assessment,* crackles and rhonchi were heard over all lung fields, and it was time to begin vigorous bronchial hygiene with bronchodilators and mucolytic agents. Because of the fear of atelectasis, hyperinflation therapy in the form of positive end-expiratory pressure (PEEP) on the ventilator might have been indicated. The sputum should have been cultured to see if any infectious organisms were present.

At the time of the *final assessment* (2 days later) the evidence for airways secretions was lessened, as the rhonchi could no longer be heard over the lung fields, and the small amount of sputum suctioned was clear. At this point, down-regulation of bronchial hygiene therapy would be indicated.

Serial FVC, FEV_1, or NIF measurements should continue to be made until such time as the patient is able to be extubated. This, indeed, happened about 3 weeks after the initiation of mechanical ventilation.

CHAPTER **25** Myasthenia Gravis

S: N/A (patient is intubated)

O: No spontaneous ventilations. Vital signs: BP 132/86, HR 90. Normal bronchial vesicular breath sounds over the right lung. Diminished-to-absent breath sounds over the left lung. ABGs: pH 7.28, $Paco_2$ 58, HCO_3^- 24, Pao_2 52. Spo_2: 80%.

A: • Endotracheal tube placed in right main stem bronchi (diminished-to-absent breath sounds over left lung, ABGs)
• Acute ventilatory failure with mild hypoxemia (ABGs)
  • Likely caused by misplacement of endotracheal tube

P: Notify physician stat. Check CXR. Pull endotracheal tube back. Monitor and reevaluate immediately.

S: N/A (patient intubated on ventilator)

O: Vital signs: BP 123/75, HR 74, T normal. Normal bronchovesicular breath sounds over both lung fields. CXR: endotracheal tube in good position; lungs adequately ventilated. ABGs: pH 7.53, $Paco_2$ 27, HCO_3^- 22, Pao_2 176. Spo_2: 98%.

A: • Acute ventilator-induced alveolar hyperventilation with overly corrected hypoxemia (ABGs)

P: Adjust present mechanical ventilation setting (e.g., decrease tidal volume). Down-regulate oxygen therapy per protocol. Monitor and reevaluate.

S: N/A

O: No improvement seen in muscular paralysis. Skin: pale. Vital signs: BP 146/88, HR 92, T 37.9° C (100.2° F). Large amounts of thick, yellowish sputum. Rhonchi over both lung fields. CXR: pneumonia and atelectasis in right lower lobe. ABGs: pH 7.28, $Paco_2$ 36, HCO_3^- 17, Pao_2 41. Spo_2: 69%.

A: • Excessive bronchial secretions (rhonchi, sputum)
  • Infection likely (yellow sputum, fever, CXR: pneumonia)
• Metabolic acidosis with moderate-to-severe hypoxemia (ABGs)
  • Likely caused by lactic acid (ABGs)

P: Start vigorous bronchial hygiene therapy per protocol (sputum culture). Hyperinflation therapy per protocol (e.g., positive end-expiratory pressure [PEEP]). Increase Fio_2 per protocol. Monitor closely and reevaluate (e.g., in 30 minutes)

Discussion

Like the case of Guillain-Barré syndrome, this case of myasthenia gravis gives us yet another chance to discuss a problem of ventilatory pump failure secondary to neuromuscular disease. The presentation of this patient with diplopia, dysphagia, and progressive muscle weakness is classic for this condition. The positive Tensilon test noted in the history is necessary for a final diagnosis. It is also important to note that it is not uncommon for these patients to aspirate gastric contents.

In the *first assessment* the reader should have picked up on the fact that this is more than simple respiratory pump failure. The reader should have seen that the patient had been intubated recently and that breath sounds were no longer present in the entire left lung (inadvertent right main stem bronchus intubation). The reader should have confirmed his or her impression with a chest x-ray film and (very quickly) pulled the endotracheal tube back and rechecked its new placement with another x-ray film. At this point, oxygenating the patient is of primary importance. Increasing the F_{IO_2} to between 0.80 and 1.0 is appropriate. One **should not** be interested in proceeding with any attempt at weaning at this early junction.

The *second assessment* should reflect the fact that the patient is improving and is now hyperventilated and hyperoxygenated on the current ventilator settings. The therapist should adjust the ventilator therapy accordingly and begin the process of longitudinal evaluation of forced vital capacity, forced expiratory volume in 1 second, and negative inspiratory force that is appropriate for this condition if weaning is to be successfully accomplished.

The *final assessment* suggests that the patient has taken another downturn. The sputum is now purulent; rhonchi are heard over both lung fields; and a right lower lobe pneumonia or atelectasis has developed. The patient now has an uncompensated metabolic acidemia that needs evaluation.

The reader should have anticipated this, obtained appropriate cultures, and if not done before, prophylactically started bronchial hygiene with frequent suctioning, percussion and postural drainage, and possibly mucolytics. The metabolic acidemia is out of proportion to the patient's condition as described. The reader may wish to review other causes of metabolic acidemia at this time (diabetic ketoacidosis, renal failure, etc.).

Unfortunately the patient's pulmonary condition progressively deteriorated, and she died 3 weeks later.

CHAPTER **26** Sleep Apnea

RESPONSE 1

S: "I'm breathing okay."

O: History: Strongly suggests obstructive sleep apnea: severe morning headaches, fatigued, irritable, excessive snoring, thrashing about in bed, depression, impotence, obesity, and ABGs. Skin: flushed and cyanotic. Distended neck veins and 4+ edema of feet and ankles to midcalf. Vital signs: BP 194/118, HR 78, RR 22, T normal. Oropharyngeal exam typical for obstructive sleep apnea. Diminished breath sounds, likely due to obesity. CXR: cor pulmonale; the lungs appeared normal. ABGs (on room air): pH 7.54, $Paco_2$ 58, HCO_3^- 39, Pao_2 52. Spo_2: 87%.

A: • Obstructive sleep apnea likely (history, cor pulmonale, ABGs, physical appearance)
• Acute alveolar hyperventilation superimposed on chronic ventilatory failure with moderate hypoxemia (ABGs)
   • Possible impending ventilatory failure

P: Oxygen therapy per protocol. If obstructive sleep apnea is confirmed, start continuous positive airway pressure (CPAP) calibration study. Monitor and reevaluate (e.g., ECG and Spo_2 every hour).

RESPONSE 2

S: "I'm breathing much better."

O: Recent diagnosis: obstructive sleep apnea—over 325 periods of apnea documented during sleep study; short muscular neck; narrow upper airway; obesity. Hct. 51%; Hb 17 g/dl. PFTs: severe restrictive disorder; sawtooth pattern was seen on the maximal inspiratory and expiratory flow-volume loops. No longer appears short of breath. Cyanotic but improved. Clear but diminished breath sounds. ABGs: pH 7.38, $Paco_2$ 82, HCO_3^- 44, Pao_2 66. Spo_2: 91%.

A: • Obstructive sleep apnea confirmed (history, polysomnographic sleep study, ABGs)
• Chronic ventilatory failure with mild hypoxemia.

P: Oxygenation therapy per protocol. Request CPAP calibration study. Ensure that patient sleeps in the head-up position or avoids sleeping on his back. Nutrition service to consult regarding slow weight loss program. Monitor and reevaluate.

Discussion

Although the diagnosis of obstructive sleep apnea is most frequently made in the outpatient setting, recent experience has shown that it often may be diagnosed in the course of an acute hospitalization as well. In the present case, although the patient was first seen in the emergency room, it soon became clear that he was ill enough to be admitted, and his workup proceeded from there.

In the *first assessment* the therapist must perform a careful examination of the patient's nasopharynx and oropharynx, as well as his chest. The typical anatomy of obstructive sleep apnea was seen. While the patient's polysomnogram and CPAP titration study were in progress, the therapist appropriately assured the patient's oxygenation (probably by use of a Venturi oxygen mask) to prevent alveolar hypoventilation. In a patient with as classic a case as this, a split night study (half standard polysomnography, half CPAP titration) may have been ordered.

The patient's neck vein distension, polycythemia, cardiomegaly, and peripheral edema all suggest cor pulmonale. This condition will improve once the patient's overall hypoventilation is treated. Many physicians would go ahead and give the patient a bicarbonate-losing diuretic, watching for worsening of metabolic acidosis while this is being done. The therapist (in this first assessment) correctly analyzes the situation as being potentially hazardous, and his or her assessment includes impending ventilatory failure, which is a real possibility.

After the *second assessment* the diagnosis has been made. Pulmonary function tests have shown upper airways obstruction and a restrictive disorder. The therapist makes sure a chest x-ray film is taken to rule out any other significant pulmonary condition. None is found. The patient's P_{CO_2}, however, has worsened, and the therapist is left to make some choices regarding treatment. The therapist elects to have the patient not sleep on his back or to sleep in the head-up position. He appropriately decides that another chest x-ray film would be in order and begins volume expansion therapy to treat the atelectasis that almost certainly is present. He suggests a nutrition consult, since the patient needs to be on a drastic weight loss program. Some clinicians would select a trial of a debuffering agent, such as acetazolamide (Diamox), to reduce the patient's bicarbonate. Others may even try respiratory stimulators, such as doxapram (Dopram), at this time.

At the end of this case the patient is still not markedly improved and still awaits the benefits of CPAP therapy. Indeed the CPAP therapy was eventually helpful. The patient had a 9 kg (20 lb) diuresis during the first week of its use, and good oxygenation was achieved with 10 cm H_2O CPAP pressure.

A diagnosis of obstructive sleep apnea can often complicate other primary respiratory disorders, such as COPD, pneumonia, atelectasis, or chest wall deformity. In these settings the care is more complicated and, if anything, should be even more data driven by careful examination of all subjective and objective data.

CHAPTER **27** Near Drowning

S: N/A (patient semicomatose, intubated on ventilator)

O: Near drowning diagnosis. Vital signs: BP 137/89, HR 122, RR 28, T 32.3° C (90.3° F). Crackles and dull percussion notes over the right and left lower lobes. Bilateral infiltrates in the lower lobes. ABGs: pH 7.23, $Paco_2$ 51, HCO_3^- 19, Pao_2 54. Spo_2: 84%.

A: • Near drowning (history)
• Pulmonary edema likely (history, crackles, infiltrates)
• Acute ventilatory failure with moderate hypoxemia (ABGs)
  • Combined metabolic and respiratory acidemia (ABGs)
  • Inadequate mechanical ventilation

P: Hyperinflation therapy per protocol (e.g., positive end-expiratory pressure [PEEP]). Adjust mechanical ventilation therapy per protocol (e.g., increase tidal volume or rate to blow off more CO_2). Increase Fio_2. Monitor and reevaluate (e.g., in 30 minutes). Repeat CXR in 2 to 4 hours.

S: N/A (patient intubated on ventilator)

O: Near drowning diagnosis. Vital signs: BP 125/86, HR 130, T 33.4° C (92.3° F). Crackles, rhonchi, and dull percussion notes over the right and left lung fields. Frothy, white sputum. ABGs: pH 7.53, $Paco_2$ 28, HCO_3^- 21, Pao_2 56. Spo_2: 89%.

A: • Near drowning (history)
• Pulmonary edema worsening (history, crackles, rhonchi, infiltrates shown in recent CXR)
  • Possible early ARDS
• Excessive bronchial secretions (rhonchi, frothy, white sputum)
• Acute ventilator-induced alveolar hyperventilation with moderate hypoxemia (ABGs)
  • Excessive mechanical ventilation

P: Up-regulate hyperinflation therapy per protocol. Down-regulate mechanical ventilation therapy per protocol (e.g., decrease tidal volume to retain more CO_2). Up-regulate oxygen therapy per protocol. Bronchial hygiene therapy per protocol. Monitor and reevaluate.

S: N/A (patient sedated, intubated on ventilator)

O: Vital signs: BP 100/60, HR 150, T 39.5° C (103° F). Cyanotic and cool. Pupils: fixed and dilated. Crackles and rhonchi over both lung fields worsening. Excessive, frothy, pink secretions in endotracheal tube. CXR: fluffy infiltrates consistent with a pulmonary edema pattern. ABGs: pH 7.35, $Paco_2$ 37, HCO_3^- 23, Pao_2 47. Spo_2: 80%.

A: • Near drowning (history)
• Pulmonary edema worsening (history, crackles, rhonchi, infiltrates shown in recent CXR)
  • Possible ARDS
• Excessive bronchial secretions (rhonchi, frothy, pinkish white sputum)
• Normal acid-base status with moderate-to-severe hypoxemia (ABGs)

P: Up-regulate hyperinflation therapy per protocol (if possible). Up-regulate oxygen therapy per protocol (if possible). Up-regulate bronchial hygiene therapy per protocol (obtain sputum for Gram stain and culture). Monitor and reevaluate.

Discussion

Respiratory care of the near drowning victim divides itself nicely into initial and supportive care. The *initial assessment* should determine that no foreign material is obstructing the upper airway and that voluntary ventilatory efforts are being made by the patient. In this case both these items were assessed and cared for in the field, and mechanical ventilation had been started.

The second phase of management of the near drowning victim consists of intelligent management of the ventilator, as it is used first to treat the pulmonary edema that almost always accompanies the near drowning episode and is used later to give support during the often ensuing ARDS-like picture. This case demonstrates all of this quite nicely.

In the *first assessment* we see that the patient is inadequately ventilated and oxygenated and that the ventilator settings have not been modified to include PEEP. All these steps are certainly indicated. It is assumed that vigorous tracheobronchial suctioning has been done up through the first assessment. If not and if the reader listed bronchial hygiene per protocol as a treatment, it is certainly not incorrect as long as it is suggested that vigorous tracheobronchial suctioning should be performed. The practitioner's observation of dullness to percussion and crackles at the bases suggests that pulmonary edema is occurring, as do the bilateral patchy infiltrates noted. Some physicians would already have bronchoscoped this patient to ensure that no foreign material was in the airways.

In the *second assessment* the patient is being successfully mechanically ventilated and is now taking at least 30 assisted breaths per minute. It would be wise to switch him to intermittent mandatory ventilation (IMV) mode at this juncture to prevent the alveolar hyperventilation that is clearly occurring. Further adjustment of the ventilator to improve his oxygenation by increasing the tidal volume or F_{IO_2} may be indicated, as may an increase in the ventilator PEEP setting. The patient now has frothy, white sputum, and vigorous bronchial hygiene is certainly indicated.

In the *last assessment* we see that the patient has tachycardia, rapid respiratory rate, and core temperature elevation to 39.5° C (103° F). This would indicate either CNS damage or pulmonary infection. The therapist should now move quickly to assess for the infection with a sputum Gram stain and culture, despite the fact that the secretions themselves are the frothy, pinkish white of pulmonary edema sputum. The patient is still hypoxemic, and his blood gases are beginning to look more and more like ARDS. If the patient is already on an F_{IO_2} of 100%, alternative forms of mechanical ventilation, such as inverse ratio ventilation, might be considered. High PEEP pressures may be necessary, as may high mean airway pressures, and the alert reader will have recognized this potential and had material at hand for emergency chest tube placement.

Two days after admission the patient died.

CHAPTER **28** Smoke Inhalation and Thermal Injuries

RESPONSE 1

S: N/A (patient comatose, intubated on ventilator)

O: Comatose. Vital signs: BP 157/105, HR 112, no spontaneous ventilations. Nasal hairs singed. Cannot assess oropharynx (patient intubated orally). Skin: cherry red. Frothy and sooty sputum. Crackles and rhonchi over both lung fields. CXR: bilateral pulmonary infiltrates consistent with pulmonary edema. ABGs: pH 7.52, $Paco_2$ 28, HCO_3^- 22, Pao_2 202. COHb: 30%. Spo_2: 98%.

A: • Smoke inhalation with extensive body burns
• Pulmonary edema (CXR, frothy sputum)
• Carbon monoxide poisoning (COHb 30%)
  • Impaired oxygen transport system
• Acute ventilator-induced alveolar hyperventilation with excessively corrected hypoxemia. Spo_2 is misleading because of COHb (ABGs, COHb)
  • Excessive mechanical ventilation

P: Up-regulate hyperinflation therapy per protocol. Bronchial hygiene therapy per protocol. Adjust mechanical ventilation per protocol to correct acute alveolar hyperventilation (e.g., decrease tidal volume or rate to retain more CO_2). Continue oxygen therapy per protocol until COHb is reduced. Contact physician to consider hyperbaric oxygen (HBO) treatments. Monitor and reevaluate (e.g., in 30 minutes).

RESPONSE 2

S: N/A (patient comatose, intubated on ventilator)

O: Skin: still cherry red. Vital signs: BP 127/88, HR 82, RR on A/C ventilation 30/min. Hemodynamics: All parameters normal. Frothy, sooty bronchial secretions. Crackles and rhonchi auscultated over both lung fields worsening. CXR: good endotracheal tube placement, pulmonary infiltrates worsening. ABGs: pH 7.29, $Paco_2$ 37, HCO_3^- 18, Pao_2 63. COHb: 20%.

A: • Pulmonary edema (CXR, frothy sputum)
• Carbon monoxide poisoning (COHb 20%)
  • Impaired oxygen transport system
• Metabolic acidosis with mild hypoxemia (ABGs and COHb)

P: Continue mechanical ventilation per protocol. Up-regulate hyperinflation therapy per protocol (e.g., increase positive end-expiratory pressure [PEEP]). Up-regulate bronchial hygiene therapy per protocol (e.g., add mucolytic, try ultrasonic nebulizer [USN], obtain sputum Gram stain and culture). Up-regulate oxygen therapy per protocol (if possible). Monitor and reevaluate (e.g., in 30 minutes).

RESPONSE 3

S: N/A (conscious but sedated, intubated, and on mechanical ventilation)

O: Excessive thick, gray and yellow secretions. Sputum culture: *Pseudomonas.* CXR: greater opacity throughout both lung fields; severe pulmonary edema, atelectasis, and ARDS. Bronchoscopy: numerous eschars and mucus plugs were suctioned. Skin: no longer red. Hemodynamics: normal. ABGs: pH 7.25, $Paco_2$ 39, HCO_3^- 18, Pao_2 37. COHb: 10%.

A: • Pulmonary edema, atelectasis, and ARDS (CXR)
 • Carbon monoxide poisoning improving (COHb 10%)
 • Metabolic acidosis with severe hypoxemia worsening (ABGs)

P: Up-regulate hyperinflation therapy per protocol (if possible). Up-regulate bronchial hygiene therapy per protocol. Up-regulate oxygen therapy per protocol. Contact physician: consider repeat therapeutic bronchoscopy. Assist in transferring patient for HBO treatment. Monitor and reevaluate (e.g., per shift).

Discussion

The patient with smoke inhalation or thermal injuries of the lung is a great challenge to the respiratory care professional. Initially, attention must be given to the upper airway, where one must ascertain if the airway is obstructed by edema secondary to the thermal burn, by the burn itself, or by foreign material obstructing the airway. Once this is known and the patient is intubated, careful respiratory care is mandatory, since severe thermal injuries to the lung are usual in most such patients, and in many of them ARDS develops.

In the *first assessment* a careful examination of the upper airway is necessary. The reader should conclude that the cherry red skin and the severe carboxyhemoglobinemia are related and that they may account for the persistence of the patient's comatose state even after he has been intubated and placed on a ventilator. In the first assessment it appears that the patient is hyperoxygenated and hyperventilated. His pulse oximeter is giving falsely high values, not correcting for the carboxyhemoglobinemia. The therapist's suggestion to increase PEEP or the F_{IO_2} or both and to reduce the assist/control rate or tidal volume or both on the ventilator are appropriate. Arrangements should be made to have this patient taken to the HBO therapy unit as soon as possible, given the dangerously high carbon monoxide levels noted. The fact that the patient has sooty-appearing sputum almost certainly indicates that the airway and lungs have severe thermal burns. This is confirmed by the pulmonary edema–like pattern seen on the chest x-ray film.

At the *second assessment* the alert reader will conclude that the patient's acid-base status is worse, with metabolic acidosis as well as mild hypoxemia. The patient's carboxyhemoglobinemia, while now improved, is still clearly an issue. The suggestion to repeat HBO therapy is appropriate. If the reader recalled that the patient's sputum culture had not yet been obtained, he or she is absolutely correct, and ordering it is appropriate. Mucolytics must be administered cautiously in this setting, since a substance such as acetylcysteine may further irritate or burn the already inflamed airway. A trial of in-line USN therapy may sooth the airway and liquefy secretions just as well.

With the *last assessment* we see that obtaining a culture was well worth while, since *Pseudomonas* organisms were identified. These will be treated appropriately with intravenous antibiotics. The fact that the pulmonary edema is not clearing suggests that the patient is developing ARDS and should suggest to the therapist that he or she is in for a long haul. Vigorous bronchial hygiene needs to continue, since eschars and mucus plugs were removed at bronchoscopy. Repeat therapeutic bronchoscopy may be indicated. The patient continues to have metabolic acidemia, the exact cause of which should be ascertained. Because the patient's Pa_{O_2} is so low, a repeat of HBO therapy is indicated, despite the fact that the patient falls below the usual institution COHb cutoff line of 10%.

The patient died 3 days after admission.

CHAPTER **29**   Postoperative Atelectasis

S: "My gut really hurts, and I can't seem to get any air."

O: Respiratory distress. Cyanotic. Vital signs: BP 185/140, HR 130, RR 35, T normal. Tachypnea. Frequent spontaneous, weak cough with yellow sputum production. LLL: diminished breath sounds; RLL, bronchial breath sounds and dull percussion notes. Incentive spirometry (IS): 40% preoperative value. Spo_2 (2 L/min O_2 nc): 77%. ABGs: pH 7.57, $Paco_2$ 23, HCO_3^- 21, Pao_2 43.

A: • Labored breathing (general appearance, vital signs, ABGs)
  • Excessive yellow sputum accumulation (sputum)
    • Possible infection
  • Weak cough effort (observation)
  • Possible atelectasis or consolidation or both in RLL (dull percussion, bronchial breath sound, IS values)
  • Acute alveolar hyperventilation with moderate-to-severe hypoxemia (ABGs)

P: Oxygenation therapy per protocol. Bronchial hygiene therapy per protocol. Hyperinflation therapy per protocol. Obtain sputum for culture. Contact physician to discuss patient status. Request chest x-ray film. Consider transfer to intensive care unit. Monitor and reevaluate.

S: No response to questions

O: Respiratory distress: cyanotic, cool, and damp. Vital signs: BP 188/144, HR 135, RR 36, T 38.1° C (100.6° F). Right middle and both lower lung lobes: dull percussion notes, bronchial breath sounds, and crackles. CXR: RML, RLL, and LLL atelectasis and bronchograms. Spo_2: 72%. ABGs: pH 7.55, $Paco_2$ 29, HCO_3^- 22, Pao_2 46.

A: • Continued labored breathing (general appearance, vital signs, ABGs)
  • Sputum accumulation still excessive (cough and recent history)
  • Weak cough effort (observation)
  • RML, RLL, and LLL atelectasis (CXR, dull percussion, bronchial breath sounds)
  • Acute alveolar hyperventilation with moderate-to-severe hypoxemia (ABGs)
    • Impending ventilatory failure

P: Up-regulate oxygenation therapy per protocol. Up-regulate bronchial hygiene therapy per protocol (obtain sputum for Gram stain and culture). Up-regulate hyperinflation therapy per protocol. Contact physician to discuss patient status. Consider therapeutic bronchoscopy. Monitor and reevaluate.

S: "I think I'm dying."

O: Obvious respiratory distress. Skin cyanotic, cool, and damp. No right-sided chest excursion. Trachea deviated to the right. Vital signs: BP 192/148, HR 142, RR 20. RML and RLL: Bronchial breath sounds, crackles, and dull percussion notes. LLL: Dull percussion notes and no breath sounds. Spo_2: 62%. ABGs: pH 7.26, $Paco_2$ 53, HCO_3^- 22, Pao_2 37.

A: • Continued increased work of breathing (general appearance, vital signs)
  • Excessive sputum accumulation still likely (recent history)
  • RML and RLL atelectasis (dull percussion, bronchial breath sounds, CXR)
  • Possible LLL atelectasis (dull percussion note, CXR)
    • Likely caused by mucus plugging (no breath sounds)
  • Acute ventilatory failure with severe hypoxemia (ABGs)

P: Contact physician stat. Recommend mechanical ventilation accompanied by oxygen therapy per protocol, bronchial hygiene therapy per protocol, and hyperinflation therapy per protocol. Request chest x-ray film. Monitor and reevaluate.

Discussion

You can almost see trouble coming! By the time of the *first assessment* this overweight, tobacco-abusing woman with a chronic productive cough *before* surgery has developed postoperative atelectasis due to pain, splinting of the chest, or postoperative analgesia. The physical findings are classic for major atelectasis initially involving the right lung and associated with severe right-to-left shunt physiology, despite alveolar hyperventilation.

In the first portion of this case the diagnosis and treatment of postoperative atelectasis with IS (and failing that, intermittent positive-pressure breathing [IPPB]) is fairly straightforward. The patient's severe hypoxemia, despite alveolar hyperventilation, however, deserves careful monitoring. It is probably safe to give this patient a much higher concentration of oxygen (e.g., 50%) by a Venturi oxygen mask. However, careful attention must be paid to oximetry and blood gas analyses. If the patient were not waking up and becoming more cooperative at this point, the blood gases are severe enough to prompt consideration of intubation and mechanical ventilation at this time.

If one "SOAPs" this patient carefully, it will be noted that there is a heavy preoperative cigarette smoking history. The alert readers would have started bronchial hygiene per protocol. The diastolic hypertension, which has persisted despite analgesia, is worrisome and needs to be monitored carefully.

At the time of the *second assessment* it is clear that the patient will not or could not cooperate with deep breathing and coughing and categorically refused chest physical therapy. The blood pressure is even higher now; the heart rate is rapid; and the patient has fever as well. The fact that the patient is unresponsive raises the question of sedation overdose and of possible CO_2 retention, but the blood gases clearly rule out CO_2 retention.

On the basis of the physical findings and the chest x-ray film the therapist appropriately assesses the cause of this as right middle and lower lobe atelectasis and possible left lower lobe atelectasis. Oxygen therapy is pushed correctly by increasing the F_{IO_2} by mask therapy. However, because of the right-to-left shunt physiology involved, this may not be successful. Bronchial hygiene and bronchodilator therapy per protocols are indicated as well, with vigorous bronchodilatation, mucolysis, and consideration of therapeutic bronchoscopy. The patient's arterial blood gases are now abnormal enough to make intubation and mechanical ventilation options at this point. Sputum from deep nasotracheal suctioning or bronchoscopy should be cultured promptly, as the patient's fever most likely represents pulmonary infection.

Certainly at the time of the *final assessment* the patient must be mechanically ventilated, as she has acute respiratory acidosis and profound hypoxemia. Her bilateral atelectasis is still present and has not been improved by the treatments outlined earlier.

It should be pointed out that by the time of the *last assessment* the patient has gone beyond the usual medical boundaries. The treating therapist's desire to contact the physician immediately and prepare for semiemergent mechanical ventilation is entirely appropriate. Inflation therapy with positive end-expiratory pressure (PEEP) as part of the mechanical ventilation order would also be appropriate, since it is clear that atelectasis is the chief villain here.

Despite vigorous therapy as outlined in this case, the patient did poorly. It was 5 days before she was able to be weaned gradually from ventilator support and 2 weeks before she was able to return home. Postoperative infection and retained secretions characterized her postoperative course.

•◦ KEY POINT ANSWERS   *For Postoperative Atelectasis (DRG 101/102)*

1. **Basic Concept Formation**
    a. It would become *smaller,* collapsed in on itself.
    b. The airless lung *could not oxygenate* blood passing through it, and hypoxemia would result.
    c. *Airway obstruction* and *small tidal volume breathing* (as under fractured ribs).
    d. *Yes.* Hyperinflation therapy (IS, IPPB, positive expiratory pressure [PEP], continuous positive airway pressure [CPAP], and PEEP administration) is a key element in the prevention and treatment of atelectasis.

2. **Data Base Formation**
    a. Atelectatic areas of lung are *small* and *airless.**
    b. *Decreased $\dot{V}/\dot{Q}$ ratio,* producing *right-to-left shunt physiology* and *hypoxemia,* and *decreased lung compliance,* producing *restrictive lung function physiology* (see Fig. 1-4). A small lung is a noncompliant lung.
    c. *Yes.* The airway *lumen* is often obstructed, and *airless surrounding structures* do not readily transmit intrapleural distending forces to obstructed, small lung units.
    d. Eventually, *acute respiratory failure* will occur. There is also some evidence to support the notion that reduced cough efficiency in such patients leads to *retained secretions* and possibly to pneumonia. Atelectasis can be progressive, involving more and more lung parenchyma. A vicious circle—difficult-to-expand lung → retained secretions → more atelectasis → more retained secretions—develops and can lead (as in this case) to ventilatory insufficiency and ventilatory failure.
    e. Atelectasis unfortunately is a common postoperative complication. Operative site pain, chest wall splinting, air swallowing with distension of abdominal viscera, and failure to cough and deep breathe are all factors in the development of postoperative atelectasis. Basically, atelectasis may also result when an airway is obstructed from any cause, and air distal to the obstruction is absorbed into the pulmonary circulation. This process is accelerated when the P_{AO_2} is high and is sometimes called *absorption atelectasis.* Finally, alveolar hypoventilation from any cause may result in atelectasis, either regionally or throughout the lung. Thus atelectasis can occur in
        (1) Chest wall injuries (flail chest)
        (2) Obesity
        (3) Myasthenia gravis and Guillian-Barré syndrome
        (4) Cervical spine injuries
        (5) Under pleuritic areas of lung
        (6) Under pneumothoraces or pleural effusions
        (7) Conditions reducing pulmonary compliance such as pulmonary fibrosis, pulmonary edema, and ARDS
    f. The *goals of therapy* in patients with atelectasis are to (1) remove secretions obstructing the airways, (2) cause deep breaths and sighs, (3) remove any extrinsic compressing factors such as pleural effusion or pneumothorax, (4) maintain alveolar stability by increasing mean airway and end-expiratory pressure, and (5) oxygenate the patient.
    g. *Oxygen Therapy, Hyperinflation Therapy*, and *Bronchial Hygiene Therapy Protocols* (see p. 6) are indicated in all patients with hypoxemia resulting from excessive airway secretions and atelectasis.
        (1) *Potential adverse effects* of these protocols include the following:
            (a) *Oxygen therapy:* Absorption atelectasis (see 2.e above) and (remotely possible) cellular oxygen toxicity
            (b) *Hyperinflation therapy* (especially with IPPB and PEEP): Pulmonary barotrauma
            (c) *Bronchial hygiene:* No specific adverse effects
        (2) Appropriate monitors in atelectasis include serial inspiratory capacity (IC) or FVC measurements, *pulse oximetry,* and *ABGs* (with calculation of A–a O_2 gradient or Pa_{O_2}/F_{IO_2} ratio), *serial chest x-ray films,* and in intubated, mechanically ventilated patients, serial measuring of *static pulmonary compliance.*

---

*See color plate 30 in Des Jardins T, Burton GG: *Clinical manifestations and assessment of respiratory disease,* ed 3, St. Louis, 1995, Mosby.

3. Assessment

a. *Yes.* Her smoking history, obesity, current history of pneumonia, asthma, COPD, the site of surgery, and the length of the procedure all predispose to the development of postoperative atelectasis.

b. *Yes.* She demonstrated tachycardia and tachypnea, hypertension, findings of consolidation (dullness to percussion, bronchial breath sounds) in the right lower lobe, restrictive physiology on pulmonary function testing, and hypoxemia, all *expected clinical manifestations of atelectasis.* The presence of crackles over the RML and RLL in the *second* assessment suggested alveolar consolidation or atelectasis. Both pneumonia and atelectasis may be the cause when crackles are heard upon auscultation.

c. *Yes.* Her *shunt physiology* was reflected in oxygen-refractory hypoxemia. Her *reduced pulmonary compliance* was reflected in her rapid, shallow breathing, restrictive pulmonary function test results, and chest x-ray film.

d. Following are the clinical manifestations that indicated the severity of the condition:

   (1) On the *first* assessment her cyanosis, tachypnea, fall in FVC to 40% of preoperative volumes, and severe hypoxemia despite low-flow oxygen therapy and hyperventilation all indicate the *seriousness* of her situation.

   (2) On the *second* assessment she is unresponsive, still tachypneic, and hypoxemic. This, in our minds, indicates *worsening,* as her comatose condition precludes use of incentive spirometry. Her hypoxemia could worsen *further* if, for example, heavy-duty analgesia such as morphine sulfate were given, her pain were relieved, and her pain-mediated hyperventilation were to cease.

   (3) On the *third and last* assessment the patient has slipped into acute respiratory failure, with respiratory acidemia and even worse ABGs.

4. Application

a. Sputum induction **was not** indicated, although she had been producing yellow sputum that had not previously been cultured. If the patient is coughing productively, there is no need to induce sputum. The respiratory care practitioner was correct in sending a specimen off to the laboratory, as infection (bronchitis or pneumonia) can cause atelectasis.

b. Oxygen therapy certainly **was** indicated because of her hypoxemia.

c. Bronchial hygiene therapy **was** indicated because of her smoking history, history of productive cough, and bronchial breath sounds. Airway secretions often obstruct airways and lead to atelectasis (see 1.c above). Their prompt expectoration or removal by coughing or suctioning both prevent and treat atelectasis. This is the rationale for deep breathing and coughing (DB&C), percussion and postural drainage (PD), and therapeutic bronchoscopy.

d. *Hyperinflation therapy* certainly **was** indicated and is the core of prevention and treatment of postoperative atelectasis.

e. At the time of the last assessment, *mechanical ventilation* **was** indicated because of her severely abnormal ABGs.

f. When the patient recovered, *pulmonary rehabilitation* **was** indicated for smoking cessation education and use of inhaled bronchodilators alone, if for no other reason.
   Summary of need for therapy: We see in this patient indications for multiple therapeutic modalities. The reader should contrast this with the needs of the patient with simple pneumonia, whose chest radiograph may appear very much like this patient's.

5. Evaluation

a. The respiratory care practitioner can expect the following results and complications from his or her choice of therapeutic modalities:

   (1) *Oxygen Therapy:* Relief of the patient's hypoxemia to the extent allowed by her shunt physiology.

   (2) *Bronchial Hygiene Therapy:* Initially, increased volume of expectorated sputum, reduction in rhonchi, arrest of atelectasis.

   (3) *Hyperinflation Therapy:* Increase in IC or FVC, improvement in CXR and ABGs as atelectasis improves; arrest of atelectasis. Periodic assessment will guide the choice between IS and IPPB therapy. IS generally is better tolerated than IPPB is, and the volume-time integral is better for IS. Air swallowing and barotrauma are known complications of IPPB but not of IS.

    (4) *Mechanical Ventilation:* PEEP therapy used if hypoxemia not improved. Improved respiratory acidemia. Barotrauma is the feared complication of mechanical ventilation.

    (5) *Pulmonary Rehabilitation:* Improved bronchial hygiene. Importance of smoking cessation understood by the patient. Increased level of day-to-day functioning, activities of daily living.

  b. *Monitors* for the success or failure of each modality are as follows:

    (1) *Oxygen Therapy:* Sp_{O_2}, ABGs

    (2) *Bronchial Hygiene Therapy:* Sputum volume, chest x-ray, Sp_{O_2}, ABGs

    (3) *Hyperinflation Therapy:* IC, FVC, Sp_{O_2}, ABGs, chest x-ray film

    (4) *Mechanical Ventilation:* ABGs, Sp_{O_2}, static compliance

  c. The *upper limits* of intensity or frequency of the necessary modalities are as follows:

    (1) *Oxygen therapy:* To an F_{IO_2} of 1.0

    (2) *Bronchial Hygiene Therapy:* Deep breathing and coughing instruction or exercises can practically be done every 30 to 60 minutes. Percussion and PD will not be tolerated more often than once every 2 to 3 hours. Therapeutic bronchoscopy can be done as often as necessary, although it usually is accompanied by intubation after the second or third procedure.

    (3) *Hyperinflation Therapy:* IS or IPPB or both can be done initially every 30 to 60 minutes. IPPB is not indicated if the patient will not or cannot use IS, if the chest x-ray film documents increasing atelectasis, if DB&C and IS are unsuccessful in preventing or treating atelectasis, or if the IC is <30% of predicted normal values. PEP, CPAP, and PEEP can be done continuously.

    (4) *Mechanical Ventilation:* is done continuously. Barotrauma limits therapy.

  d. The *least invasive* of the indicated therapies for atelectasis are DB&C, IS, mask CPAP, and O_2 therapy. *More intrusive* are IPPB and bronchodilation therapy. *More expensive and invasive* and associated with known side effects or risks are therapeutic bronchoscopy, mechanical ventilation, and PEEP therapy. Despite this hierarchy of risks and costs, early use of therapeutic bronchoscopy often is ultimately cost effective, as it treats atelectasis secondary to airway obstruction at its core.

  e. If the monitors listed in 5.b above indicate *improvement,* we would discontinue mechanical ventilation and extubate the patient first, maintaining aggressive bronchial hygiene therapy and hyperinflation therapy in the form of IS for at least 3 to 4 days thereafter. Oxygen therapy would be tapered as ABGs or Sp_{O_2} volumes allow.

  f. If the patient *did not improve* (as in this case), aggressive therapeutic bronchoscopy, intubation, and mechanical ventilation with pressure support and PEEP would be indicated.

6. Boundary Awareness

  a. This patient is critically ill at the time of the *first* assessment (see 3.d above) and progressively worsens in the next two scenarios. Her ABGs, Sp_{O_2}, and chest x-ray films all point this out.

  b. Literally, at *any time* in this critically ill patient. Certainly at the time of the *third* assessment.

  c. As in 6.b above. In cases of atelectasis, it is suggested that a physician be called when the Sp_{O_2} cannot be kept above 88%, when respiratory or metabolic acidosis supravenes, when a new lobe collapses on the chest x-ray film, and whenever bronchoscopy or mechanical ventilation appears to be necessary.

RESPIRATORY ASSESSMENT FLOW CHART

Subjective →

Objective →

Vital signs: RR ___ HR ___ BP ___

Temp. ___ On antipyratic agent? ☐ Yes ☐ No

Chest assessment:

Insp. ___

Palp. ___

Perc. ___

Ausc. ___

Radiography ___

Bedside spir.: PEFR $\bar{a}$ ___ $\bar{p}$ ___ Tx ___

SVC ___ FVC ___ NIF ___

Cough: ☐ Strong ☐ Weak

Sputum production: ☐ Yes ☐ No

Sputum char. ___

ABG: pH ___ PaCO$_2$ ___ HCO$_3$ ___

PaO$_2$ ___ SaO$_2$ ___ SpO$_2$ ___

Neg. O$_2$ transport factors

Other: ___

Anterior

L

R

Posterior

R

L

Pt. name

	Male	Female
Age		
Date	Time	

Admitting diagnosis

Therapist

Hospital

Assessment →

Plan →

PRESENT PLAN

PLAN MODIFICATIONS

Index

A

Abbreviations, 9
Abscess, lung
    case study of, 61-65
    SOAP responses for, 199-200
Accident
    burn injury and
        case study of, 161-165
        SOAP responses for, 241-242
    flail chest and
        case study of, 91-95
        SOAP responses for, 211-212
    near drowning
        case study of, 155-159
        SOAP responses for, 239-240
Acquired immunodeficiency syndrome
    case study of, 57-60
    SOAP responses for, 197-198
Adult respiratory distress syndrome
    case study of, 127-131
    interrelationships in, 12
    key point answers for, 227-228
    SOAP responses for, 225-226
Airway weakening, 15
Alcohol abuse, 91
Alveolar-capillary membrane thickness, 12
Alveolar consolidation, 11
Alveolar disease, diffuse; see Diffuse
        alveolar disease
Alveolar weakening, 15
Anatomic alternations of lung, 8-15
    alveolar-capillary membrane thickness
        and, 12
    alveolar consolidation and, 11
    atelectasis and, 10
    bronchospasm and, 13
    emphysema and, 15
    excessive secretions and, 14
Apnea, sleep
    case study of, 151-154
    SOAP responses for, 237-238
Asbestosis
    case study of, 115-120
    SOAP responses for, 219-221

Assessment, therapist-driven protocols in,
        1-15; see also Therapist-driven
        protocols in assessment
Asthma
    case study of, 33-38
    interrelationships in, 13, 14
    key point answers for, 185-188
    SOAP responses for, 183-184
Atelectasis, postoperative
    case study of, 167-172
    interrelationships in, 10
    key point answers for, 245-247
    SOAP responses for, 243-244

B

Bronchial hygiene therapy protocol, 6
Bronchial secretions, excessive, 14
Bronchiectasis
    case study of, 27-31
    SOAP responses for, 181-182
Bronchitis, chronic
    case study of, 17-22
    interrelationships in, 14
    key point answers for, 177-178
    SOAP responses for, 173-175
Bronchodilator therapy protocol, 6
    bronchospasm and, 13
Bronchospasm, 13
Burn injury
    case study for, 161-165
    SOAP responses for, 241-242

C

Cancer, lung
    case study of, 121-126
    SOAP responses for, 223-224
Chest trauma
    flail chest and, 91-95
    pneumothorax and, 97-101
Chest wall disorder
    case study of, 109-114
    SOAP responses for, 217-218

Child
   asthma in, 33-38
   croup syndrome in, 45-49
   respiratory distress in, 133-136
Chronic bronchitis; *see* Bronchitis, chronic
Chronic interstitial lung disease
   case study of, 137-141
   SOAP responses for, 231-232
Coccidioidomycosis
   case study of, 73-77
   SOAP responses for, 203-204
Consolidation, alveolar, 11
Croup syndrome
   case study of, 45-49
   SOAP responses for, 191
Curvature of spine, 109-114
   SOAP responses for, 217-218
Cystic fibrosis, 39-43
   SOAP responses for, 189-190

D

Diffuse alveolar disease
   adult respiratory distress syndrome and
      case study of, 127-131
      key point answers for, 227-228
      SOAP responses for, 225-226
   infant respiratory distress syndrome and
      case study of, 133-136
      SOAP responses for, 229-230
Documentation of assessment process, 3
Drowning, near
   case study of, 155-159
   SOAP responses for, 239-240

E

Edema, pulmonary
   case study of, 79-84
   key point answers for, 207-208
   SOAP responses for, 205-206
Effusion, pleural
   case study of, 103-107
   SOAP responses for, 215-216
Embolism, pulmonary
   case study of, 85-88
   SOAP responses for, 209-210
Emphysema
   case study of, 23-26
   interrelationships in, 15
   SOAP responses for, 179-180
Environmental lung disease
   case study of, 115-120
   SOAP responses for, 219-221

F

Fibrosis, cystic
   case study of, 39-43
   SOAP responses for, 189-190
Flail chest
   case study of, 91-95
   SOAP responses for, 211-212
Fungal infection
   case study of, 73-77
   SOAP responses for, 203-204

G

Guillain Barré syndrome
   case study of, 143-146
   SOAP responses for, 233-234

H

Human immunodeficiency virus infection
   case study of, 57-60
   SOAP responses for, 197-198
Hyperinflation therapy, 6, 12
   for atelectasis, 10
Hypoxemia
   alveolar-capillary membrane thickness
      and, 12
   alveolar consolidation and, 11
   atelectasis and, 10

I

Infant respiratory distress syndrome
   case study of, 133-136
   SOAP responses for, 229-230
Infectious disease
   acquired immunodeficiency syndrome as
      case study of, 57-60
      SOAP responses for, 197-198
   fungal
      case study of, 73-77
      SOAP responses for, 203-204
   lung abscess as
      case study of, 61-65
      SOAP responses for, 199-200
   pneumonia as
      case study of, 51-56
      key point answers for, 195-196
      SOAP responses for, 193-194
   tuberculosis as
      case study of, 67-71
      SOAP responses for, 201-202
Inhalation, smoke
   case study of, 161-165
   SOAP responses for, 241-242

Interstitial lung disease
    case study of, 137-141
    SOAP responses for, 231-232

K

Knowledge base for respiratory care
      practitioner, 1-2
Kyphosis
    case study of, 109-114
    SOAP responses for, 217-218

L

Lung abscess
    case study of, 61-65
    SOAP responses for, 199-200
Lung cancer
    case study of, 121-126
    SOAP responses for, 223-224
Lung infection; *see* Infectious disease

M

Malignancy
    case study of, 121-126
    SOAP responses for, 223-224
Mechanical ventilation protocol, 13
Muscle disorder
    Guillain Barré syndrome as
      case study of, 143-146
      SOAP responses for, 233-234
    myasthenia gravis as
      case study of, 147-150
      SOAP responses for, 235-236
Myasthenia gravis
    case study of, 147-150
    SOAP responses for, 235-236

N

Near drowning
    case study of, 155-159
    SOAP responses for, 239-240
Neoplastic disease
    case study of, 121-126
    SOAP responses for, 223-224
Neurologic disorder
    Guillain Barré syndrome as
      case study of, 143-146
      SOAP responses for, 233-234
    myasthenia gravis as
      case study of, 147-150
      SOAP responses for, 235-236

O

Obstructive airway disease, 7
    asthma as
      case study of, 33-38
      interrelationships in, 13, 14
      key point answers for, 185-188
      SOAP responses for, 183-184
    bronchiectasis as
      case study of, 181-182
      SOAP responses for, 181-182
    bronchiectasis as, case study of, 27-31
    chronic bronchitis as
      case study of, 17-22
      interrelationships in, 14
      key point answers for, 177-178
      SOAP responses for, 173-175
    croup syndrome as
      case study of, 45-49
      SOAP responses for, 191
    cystic fibrosis as
      case study of, 39-43
      SOAP responses for, 189-190
    emphysema as
      case study of, 23-26
      interrelationships in, 15
      SOAP responses for, 179-180
Occupational disorder
    case study of, 115-120
    SOAP responses for, 219-221
Oxygen therapy protocol, 6
    bronchospasm and, 13
    emphysema and, 15

P

Parenchymal disease, 137-141
Pathophysiologic mechanisms in respiratory
      disorders, 8-15
    alveolar consolidation and, 11
    atelectasis and, 10
    bronchospasm and, 13
    emphysema and, 14
    excessive secretions and, 14
    increased thickness of alveolar-capillary
      membrane and, 12
Pleural disease
    case study of, 103-107
    SOAP responses for, 215-216
Pneumoconiosis
    case study of, 115-120
    SOAP responses for, 219-221
Pneumonia
    case study of, 51-56
    interrelationships in, 11

Pneumonia—cont'd
    key point answers for, 195-196
    SOAP responses for, 193-194
Pneumothorax
    case study of, 97-101
    SOAP responses for, 213-214
Postoperative atelectasis
    case study of, 167-172
    interrelationships in, 10
    key point answers for, 245-247
    SOAP responses for, 243-244
Pulmonary edema
    case study of, 79-84
    interrelationships in, 12
    key point answers for, 207-208
    SOAP responses for, 205-206
Pulmonary embolism
    case study of, 85-88
    SOAP responses for, 209-210
Pulmonary rehabilitation, 15
Pulmonary vascular disease; *see* Vascular
    disease, pulmonary

R

Respiratory distress syndrome
    adult
        case study of, 127-131
        key point answers for, 227-228
        SOAP responses for, 225-226
    infant
        case study of, 133-136
        SOAP responses for, 229-230
Restrictive respiratory disorder, 7

S

Sleep apnea
    case study of, 151-154
    SOAP responses for, 237-238
Smoke inhalation
    case study of, 161-165
    SOAP responses for, 241-242
SOAP form, 3
Spinal deformity
    case study of, 109-114
    SOAP responses for, 217-218

T

Therapist-driven protocols in assessment,
    1-15, 8
    anatomic lung alterations and, 8
    bronchodilator therapy, 13-14

Therapist-driven protocols in assessment—
    cont'd
    disorders assessed in, 7
    hyperinflation, 10, 12
    knowledge base in, 1, 2
    no specific care, 11
    pulmonary rehabilitation, 15
    respiratory care, 3-4
    treatment protocols and, 4-6
Thermal injury
    case study of, 161-165
    SOAP responses for, 241-242
Trauma
    burn injury and
        case study of, 161-165
        SOAP responses for, 241-242
    flail chest and
        case study of, 91-95
        SOAP responses for, 211-212
    pneumothorax and
        case study of, 97-101
        SOAP responses for, 213-214
Treatment protocols, 4-7
Tuberculosis
    case study of, 67-71
    SOAP responses for, 201-202
Tumor
    case study of, 121-126
    SOAP responses for, 223-224

V

Vascular disease, pulmonary
    pulmonary edema as
        case study of, 79-84
        key point answers for, 207-208
        SOAP responses for, 205-206
    pulmonary embolism as
        case study of, 85-88
        SOAP responses for, 209-210
Virus infection, human immunodeficiency
    case study of, 57-60
    SOAP responses for, 197-198

W

Weakening, airway and alveolar, 15
Weakness, muscle
    Guillain Barré syndrome and
        case study of, 143-146
        SOAP responses for, 233-234
    myasthenia gravis and
        case study of, 147-150
        SOAP responses for, 235-236